RADICAL LIFE EXTENSION

Praise for *Radical Life Extension*

Easily the best introduction to the science behind the technologies that are poised to overcome the biological limits to human lifespan.

—Nathan Cheng, Co-Founder of the *Longevity Biotech Fellowship*

This book provides an accessible and wide-ranging exploration of aging and the technologies that may influence its future. It succeeds in bringing cutting-edge scientific ideas to a broader audience while encouraging discussion about longevity research.

—Steve Horvath, Professor, developer of the epigenetic clock

Death is humanity's greatest unsolved problem, and this book refuses to treat it as inevitable. It is a thoughtful call to action for anyone who believes that saving lives on a massive scale should be our highest priority.

—Adam Gries, Co-Founder of *Vitalism*

Biostasis does not guarantee anything, but cremation guarantees that you are dead forever. This book makes a compelling case for Human Biostasis as a chance when today's medicine has reached its limits.

—Emil Kendziorra, CEO of *Tomorrow Biostasis*

This book takes a properly hard-nosed view of longevity science, focusing on damage accumulation rather than getting lost in mechanistic minutiae. It's a rather refreshing reminder that solving aging is, at heart, an engineering challenge.

—Aubrey de Grey, author of *Ending Aging*

Radical Life Extension

Technological Strategies to Defeat Aging

Kristopher A. Borer

Radical Life Extension
Kristopher A. Borer

Keywords: aging, bioengineering, biostasis, cryonics, longevity, replacement

Version: 20260624
First published July 6th, 2026

ISBNs
paperback: 978-1-951974-05-3
hardcover: 978-1-951974-06-0
ebook: 978-1-951974-07-7
audiobook: 978-1-951974-08-4

Library of Congress Control Number: 2026901362

Written using the Vim text editor (vim.org)
Cover created with GIMP (gimp.org)
Print layout done with Scribus (scribus.net)
Ebook generated with Calibre (calibre-ebook.com)

krisborer.com

to Lyra

Contents

INTRODUCTION

When I was 18 years old, I realized I was going to die.

I was lying in bed in my college dorm thinking about the universe: very large, very old, and likely to endure for an unimaginably long time. Eventually, it will disappear, which is sad. But long before that, I will disappear, and that is terrifying.

There is something special about experiencing mortal terror. Normally, we are so good at ignoring our own mortality. It's easy to focus on the here and now, the latest news or pressing problems. Yet, every once in a while, my thoughts slip through the protective barriers and, briefly, I notice my dire circumstances.

I don't enjoy it, but I've found that an occasional reminder helps put things in perspective. What should I be doing with my life that is both urgent and important? It helps make clear what is not worth worrying about or getting upset about. It's much easier to forgive and forget the minor insults and conflicts of everyday life when you view them in light of life's brevity.

More recently, I discovered that there is a nascent but serious scientific effort to cure aging. Much is now understood about why and how we age, and credible strategies are in development to slow or reverse it. I became convinced enough of their potential to invest my own money into companies pursuing them, which gave me an unusually close view of both the technologies and the people building them. While this book does not recommend any specific product or company, it does use these insights to help highlight the most promising areas of research and development.

I am under no illusions: these technologies are far from ready. Yet, there is ample opportunity to accelerate their arrival.

This book is for those who want to do just that—develop technology that could extend human lifespan far beyond its current limits. For malcontents who think 100 or even 120 years is not nearly enough time to do everything they want to do. For iconoclasts who aim to really save lives, not just eke out a few extra years.

Radical life extension would be a profound good for the world, but this book is not intended to convince you of that. It is written for those who are already driven to develop longevity technology, and therefore focuses more on the how than the why.

There is no simple answer. No silver bullet or weird trick. Surprisingly, the answer depends on who you are, how much time you have left, and how much risk you are willing to take. The chapters that follow examine why aging happens, why most proposed interventions are unlikely to be enough, and why three categories of technology—biostasis, replacement, and bioengineering—may matter most.

Furthermore, this book omits anything not essential to the mission. No supplement recommendations or fad diets. No hype or false hope. The goal is to give you a clear view of where medical technology is, and where it might need to go to solve aging.

I hope that this book will elucidate both the challenges and the opportunities in the field. I also hope that once you understand them, you will join those of us working to solve aging. If you decide to, then let me thank you in advance. We have a lot to do.

Kris Borer

July 6, 2026

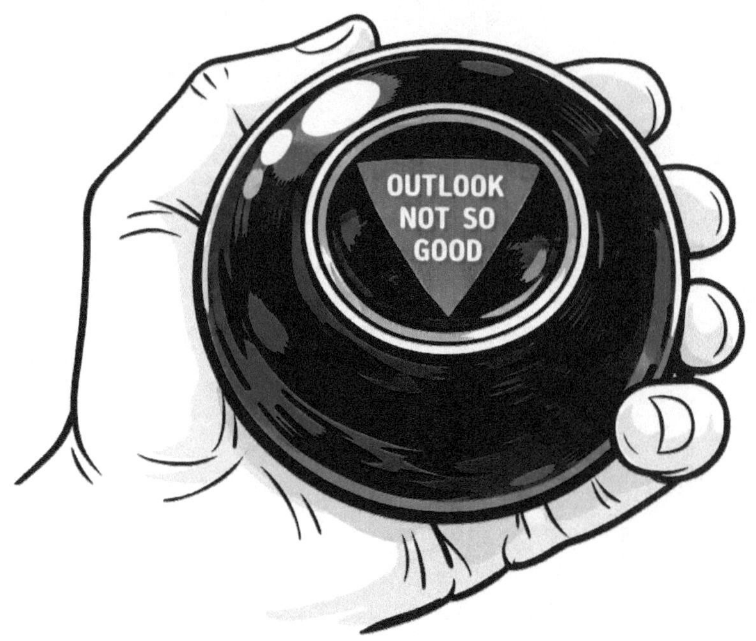

OUTLOOK
NOT SO
GOOD

CHAPTER 1

THE CURRENT SITUATION

Death should be optional.

Unfortunately, if you live a normal life, you will eventually die. Over time, the human body breaks down like any other machine. Your body can repair itself, but there are types of damage it can't fix. This damage accumulates, which is why most people live less than a century, and nobody survives to their 125th birthday.

Your lifespan is shaped by your genes, your environment, and your choices, so you do have some control over how long you live. If you eat well and exercise, you'll probably live a bit longer. However, no diet or exercise routine will keep you going forever.

Then again, there's no fundamental reason humans couldn't enjoy much longer lives. In principle, every disease has a technical solution. Developing these technologies is an ongoing process, from vaccines and antibiotics to cell therapies and gene editing. With today's technology, people already live longer than they once did. With future technologies, people may have the opportunity to live as long as they choose.

When that time will arrive is uncertain. What is certain is that what you do with the rest of your natural life will affect your chances of being around when it does. For many people alive today, reaching that future will take more than a healthy lifestyle. It will require technologies that add decades to their lives. In the long run, advanced technology is the only thing that can keep you out of the grave.

Fortunately, everyone can contribute to developing radical life extension technology. How you can best do so depends on who you are, but simply being involved is enough to make an impact. Regardless of your circumstances, the path forward will require hard work, ingenuity, and help from others. Others will need your help as well. No single person could develop the technology and infrastructure required to sustain life indefinitely, but together we can.

The sooner that time arrives, the more people can be saved. Moreover, it doesn't take much to make a difference. On the order of 150,000 people die every day. If your personal contribution to the longevity field can accelerate progress by even a single second, you will save someone. Not an abstract statistic, but a living person who would otherwise be lost.

Sadly, this also means that over 100 people died while you were reading this chapter. This is an emergency, and every second counts.

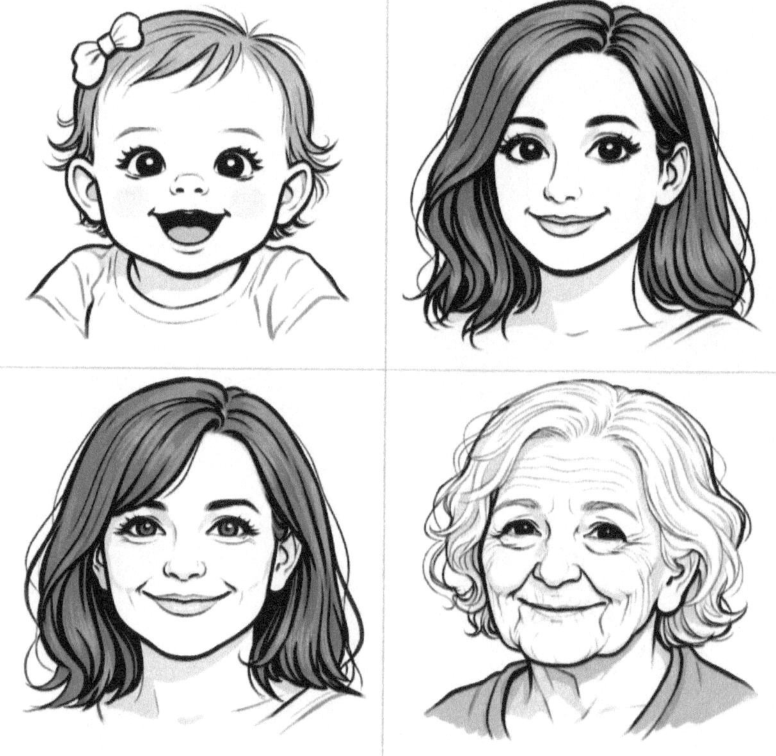

CHAPTER 2

AGING

Many things can kill you, but in the modern world the most likely one is aging. Aging is the main reason hearts stop beating, cells become cancerous, and brains degenerate. If you slow aging, you will delay the onset of strokes, tumors, and dementias. If you can reverse aging, they may never happen at all.

Slowing or reversing aging is arduous, so if your goal is merely to be relatively healthy for your age and live a little longer than expected, then it doesn't make much sense to worry about aging per se. There are plenty of scientifically proven methods for marginal life extension and a plethora of books that will tell you all about them.

However, if you want to greatly extend human lifespan, then aging is the most important thing to work on. There are several strategies for treating aging but, to take advantage of them, you will need to understand what aging is.

Aging isn't a single process, but an emergent property of a complex collection of changes to your body. A useful definition has to be abstract enough to cover all the essential changes, yet specific enough to exclude things that are merely byproducts of aging.

First, we know that aging is associated with physical changes to the body. Children also change over time, but they grow and become more robust instead of withering away. So, a second feature of aging is functional decline: an aged adult is slower, weaker, and more vulnerable. However, this also happens when someone has an infection. The difference is that infections usually pass after a while, but aging doesn't. Therefore, a third property of aging is that it doesn't get resolved, but instead becomes worse over time. Depending on circumstances, a person might temporarily appear a little younger than expected but, in the long run, age-related decline is not only inexorable, but the best we can hope for. Nobody dies suddenly of old age, so a fourth characteristic of aging is that it happens slowly. Adults don't visibly age from one day to the next, but a 30-year absence makes the physical toll of time unmistakable.

There are many things that kill us more quickly than old age, but they usually attack a specific part of the body. Snake venom can prevent your heart from beating. Aging, by contrast, degrades every part of the body. So a fifth feature of aging is that it occurs throughout the entire body. While it isn't uniform in all tissues, we would not expect half of someone's body to age while the other half stays young, nor are there any organs or tissues that completely escape age-related decline.

Not only is aging diffuse throughout the body, it's also highly varied. The way aging damages your eyes is different from how it damages your lungs. So a sixth feature of aging is that it isn't a single problem, but the combination of a large number of contributing factors. We know that some of these factors are intrinsic to human life because we age regardless of where we live or what we do. Lifestyle can affect the rate of aging but, for us, aging is a natural part of life. Other factors are external, such as the effect of air pollution on lifespan. Lucky genes might keep you younger for longer, and an unhealthy environment will age you faster.

In short, aging is the gradual accumulation of many small changes, driven by both intrinsic biology and external factors, that together cause the whole body to decline in function. At the biochemical level, it's a diverse set of processes that slowly and continuously degrade tissues throughout the body. The effect is clear, but what underlying changes produce the outward signs of aging? Which specific shifts inside our bodies create the stark contrast between someone at 25 and the same person at 75?

Underlying Mechanisms

Molecules in our bodies are always changing. Sometimes this is part of normal biological processes, such as storing and using fat reserves. Other times molecular change is a side effect, like when your body creates a scar instead of fully healing a wound. Changes also come from external factors like harmful germs, pollution, and sunlight. Even the food we eat and the air we breathe can change our bodies over time.

Molecular change isn't inherently bad. Growing taller and stronger during puberty is very different from the brain shrinkage and muscle wasting that occur in old age. Aging isn't just change, but change that eventually leads to disease and death. For example, dozens of times per day the DNA in a typical human cell breaks at some point along its length. The cell has proteins that repair these double-strand breaks, but occasionally the cell makes a mistake that changes its genetic sequence.

Most of the time random DNA mutations will have no effect, because human cells are highly tolerant of point mutations other than in a few critical locations, so changes in the vast majority of a cell's DNA won't impact its function. It's even possible for such a mutation to improve the function of a cell, but this is extremely rare. DNA mutations are more likely to have a negative impact on cell function than a positive one by corrupting the sequence a gene needs to do its job.

These negative changes are the ones that matter for aging. Detrimental change can be referred to as damage, and detrimental changes associated with aging can be called aging damage. Most molecular changes aren't damage, but even the ones that are don't necessarily cause aging because they are repaired by the body and have no long-term impact. A paper cut eventually heals but, to produce a lasting effect like aging, the damage must stick around. Your body experiences transient damage all the time, but it's mostly able to restore things. For example, we don't usually need to worry about insect bites or minor burns.

If our bodies were able to repair all damage, we would not age. Our bodies would change according to developmental programs, but then we would remain in young adulthood. You could still die in a car accident, but any minor injuries or infections would heal completely and not result in aging.

Humans do have relatively good damage repair mechanisms, which is part of why we live so long compared to most other animals. Your body is equipped to handle many types of damage, so even if random problems occur, the damage often doesn't accumulate over time. Biologists refer to this self-regulating recovery as homeostasis; unfortunately, in humans, this system is imperfect. There are many types of damage that our bodies can't fix, like DNA mutations. The damage we can't repair builds over time, eventually impairing our normal homeostatic abilities and leading to a cascade of system failures terminating in death.

Interestingly, the types of damage that our bodies can repair change over time. Children up to the age of 11 can regrow fingertips that have been amputated, but older adults have a hard time healing superficial wounds. Another example is cellular senescence, which is a cell state that promotes inflammation and helps with healing. Senescent cells are supposed to be cleared quickly. When you're young, your body rapidly removes them. As the immune system becomes less effective in old age, senescent cell clearance happens at a slower pace, so some of them escape and build up in your tissues.

Many types of damage like this are easy for your body to fix when you're young but begin to accumulate as you age. Part of the reason is that damage impairs all bodily functions, including damage repair systems. This feedback loop means that the older you are, the faster damage accumulates and the slower it's repaired. Aging damage becomes a runaway train: the faster it goes, the harder it is to stop, and the older you are, the faster you age.

Think of aging damage as debt. When you're young, the debt is small and manageable. But as damage accumulates, the interest payments grow until they consume your entire biological budget. Once you can't pay the bills, it's lights-out.

Another example of damage that accumulates late in life but not in youth is lipofuscin. Lipofuscin is molecular waste that cells can't break down, so your cells just hold on to it. Cells can reduce the amount of lipofuscin they have by dividing, with each daughter cell getting half. So for rapidly growing organisms like children, lipofuscin damage doesn't lead to aging. Fully grown adults don't have this option so, for them, lipofuscin accumulates and leads to aging.

At the molecular level, it's almost as if Murphy's law applies: anything that can go wrong will go wrong. Lipids that usually support the cell membrane get oxidized and disrupt the barrier instead. Carbohydrates are built with the wrong branching pattern, which leads to scrambled intercellular communication. Proteins become misfolded and deactivate or become actively harmful.

Sometimes the molecules themselves don't change, but the quantities or locations are wrong. Older bodies produce less collagen, which leads to weaker skin. Harmful molecules that we're exposed to, like PCBs (polychlorinated biphenyls), build up and cause cancer. Even normally helpful molecules can be harmful, like when DNA that normally resides inside power-generating organelles called mitochondria spills out into the cell's cytoplasm, causing an immune reaction. Any change from normality can negatively impact cellular processes, organelles, cell behavior, and organ function.

In general, damage might be the alteration of something to make it dysfunctional, like when genes mutate and can't produce functional products. The loss or absence of something can be damage as well. Just as a bucket is damaged if it's missing the bottom, your body is damaged if it's missing a toe, cell, or other important piece. Similarly, the addition of things can be damage. Just as the growth of barnacles on a ship can slow it down, the buildup of plaques in arteries can lead to cardiovascular disease, and the accumulation of persistent viruses can disrupt cellular and immune function.

Looking from a molecular level, we can define aging from the perspective of underlying causes. Aging is the gradual accumulation of diverse damage throughout the body. It's this ever-growing damage burden that produces the ever-increasing problems associated with aging. It isn't a single process that can be addressed with a single drug or therapy. Aging comprises a vast array of simultaneous, detrimental changes that accumulate exponentially within the human body.

Patterns in Aging Damage

Damage is often predictable on a large scale, but unpredictable at a small scale. If your skin is exposed to ultraviolet radiation, you know that many cells in the exposed area will die from sunburn. What you don't know is which cells will be affected and what mutations will be caused in each cell. This kind of random damage can occur simply as a byproduct of metabolism—the intricate web of chemical reactions driving all of the processes of life. For example, mistakes are occasionally made during DNA replication and you never know where the mutations will occur. Metabolism also produces predictable damage, like the accumulation of disulfide bonds in the lens of your eyes, eventually contributing to farsightedness.

However, even if the exact location of damage is largely random, and there are a great number of types of damage, the problem of aging isn't completely intractable. We see consistent patterns in which types of damage happen more frequently, where they tend to occur, how detrimental they are, and how well the body is equipped to deal with them. This allows us to categorize, prioritize, and strategize.

There are different ways of categorizing aging damage, but one of the most useful is to consider different levels of abstraction. At the lowest level, damage accumulation is fundamentally molecular, and microscopic changes are what eventually lead to macroscopic problems like functional decline and disease. In the middle are age-related conditions in tissues and organs like thin skin, overactive immune cells, brittle bones, and weaker hearts. At the highest level, we see people get old visually, and we can talk about how their bodies look and behave as they age.

Detrimental changes at any level of biological function can be thought of as damage, but in aging the dysfunction we see at higher levels almost always traces back to problems at lower levels. Organs fail when their tissues malfunction, tissues fail when their cells misbehave or their connective tissue is altered, and cells misbehave because of problematic molecules in their internal or external environment. In essence, aging is ultimately due to molecular damage.

Having said that, it's useful to discuss aging at different organizational levels without always having to reference the underlying structure. You can say that immune cells becoming more inflammatory is a type of aging damage even if the underlying cause is a problem with DNA expression. You can say that a heart is aged because it lost muscle cells. You can say that a cardiovascular system is aged because the arterial walls are stiff. It would get old quick if we always had to talk about molecules, even though aging is fundamentally molecular.

The first attempt to comprehensively categorize aging damage and potential solutions was the Strategies for Engineered Negligible Senescence, published in 2002. Additional categorizations continue to emerge with slightly different viewpoints, but the main idea is the same: find ways to group aging damage to make aging easier to understand and treat. Some of the proposed categories are briefly outlined below.

Extracellular waste products are molecules that build up outside of cells, like the protein amyloid beta, which clumps up in the brain during Alzheimer's disease. Intracellular waste products are molecules that build up inside cells, such as oxidized cholesterol, which disrupts cell membranes.

Cancerous cells are cells that grow uncontrollably, forming tumors and blood cancers. Normally, cells are like puppets, controlled by regulatory strings that dictate when they should grow or die. Cancer is Pinocchio once his strings have been cut—he no longer has anything to hold him down. Death-resistant cells are cells that aren't growing uncontrollably, but aren't dying when they should. This includes senescent cells, which can no longer divide and are supposed to be cleaned up by the immune system, but instead hang around causing inflammation. Cell loss means having too few cells to keep tissues working properly, either because the stem cells that renew cell populations are lost or malfunctioning, or cells are dying faster than stem cells can replace them.

Mitochondrial dysfunction leads to decline in the capability to convert stored energy into more readily usable forms. As a result, cells have a progressively harder time doing their jobs and even just surviving.

ECM stiffening refers to chemical cross-linking of the extracellular matrix, the spongy mesh that cells produce to give shape to your organs and tissues. As the mechanical properties of the ECM change with age, a variety of health problems occur. This category is often overlooked, but is very important because aging does not only occur in cells, but also outside of them. The ECM is molecular scaffolding that cells live on and inside. It can have a variety of properties, like rigidity of the bone or flexibility of the skin. Aging of the ECM leads to bone fractures and wrinkles. ECM also affects cell behavior, so cells living on old ECM will behave incorrectly and contribute to aging.

More recent damage categorization systems have fleshed out details at every level of abstraction from molecular to systemic, broken down subcategories, and arguably added at least one category, but the basic ideas remain the same. We see common patterns in age-related damage that can help us prioritize what to work on.

Other Ways of Looking at Aging

When enough damage is done to ECM and cells, either by the slow accumulation of changes that the body can't fix, or when a threshold of fixable damage is crossed that overwhelms the repair mechanisms, the aging process accelerates. We see this in mortality risk charts like the one below.

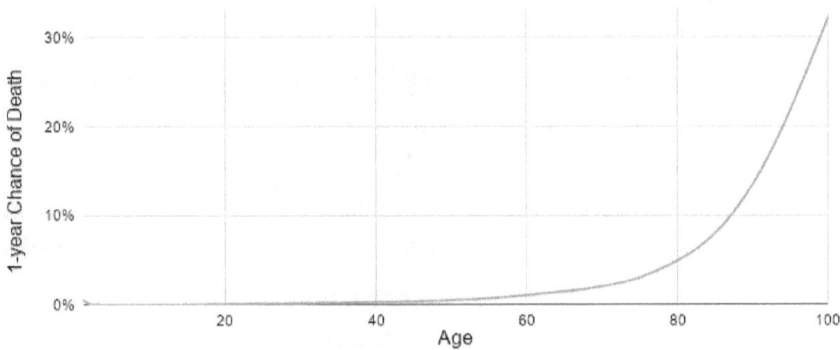

A chart showing the exponential increase in mortality risk at advanced age.

Mortality risk doesn't fully capture aging, though. Aging occurs in the young, albeit at a slower rate that's masked by developmental changes. This is because in the first decade or two of life, developmental programs have a greater influence on mortality, and the effects of aging are diluted by growth. Even though aging occurs in children, their survival rate actually increases for several years as the benefits of development outpace the detriments from aging.

Zooming in on the first 50 years makes it easier to see:

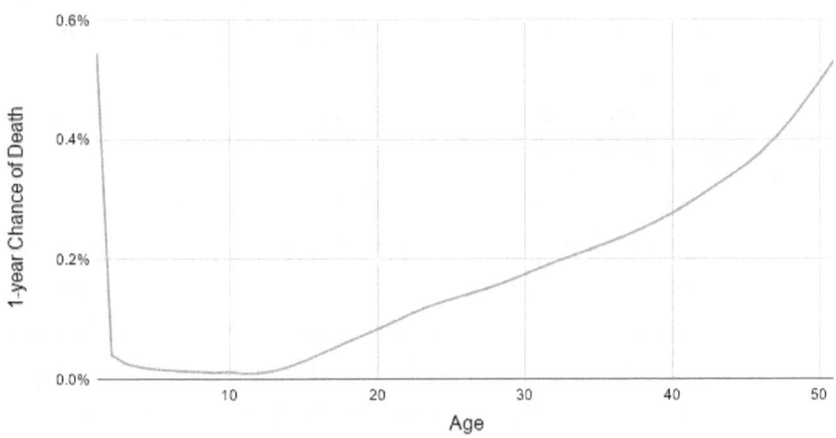

A chart showing the decreasing mortality risk from birth to adolescence.

The progression of aging is even stranger at the very beginning of life. The processes of creating eggs and sperm and developing embryos have unique and essential mechanisms to reset aging. By some measures, the early embryo actually gets younger over the first few weeks, before the balance shifts back toward aging. That's why older parents, who have damaged sperm and eggs, can still produce young, healthy babies. Unfortunately, the mechanisms involved aren't necessarily available to adults. For example, continually growing organisms can easily dilute extracellular waste products, such that they don't reach concentrations sufficient to impair function—but adults can't simply double in size to halve the concentration of garbage in their extracellular matrix.

Just like mortality risk, functional decline isn't a perfect view into the aging process. Some functional biomarkers, like maximum heart rate, have nice, smooth correlations with age. Others, such as blood pH, may see no detrimental effect until damage accumulation reaches a certain threshold. After that, the functional impact may be sudden and devastating, as with a serious stroke.

Instead of looking at one risk factor like mortality, or a handful of functional metrics, you can combine many data points into aging clocks. These are mathematical models that operate on large numbers of biomarkers and can produce a "biological age" score. Your biological age can tell you the relative amount of damage in your body. If you're 50 years old, but you score a 45, congratulations, you're healthier than the average person of your age. Conversely, if you score a 65, then something might be wrong.

While biological age scores are fun and somewhat informative, they also have important limitations. Compressing aging into a single number discards nuance: aging is the accumulation of microscopic changes that add up to macroscopic dysfunction, like when the breakdown of elastin fibers in the lungs makes it harder for the elderly to breathe. Two people with the same biological age may carry very different mixes of damage, so the abstraction can mislead about an individual's actual risks. It can also narrow thinking about how to reduce or reverse aging, because you can sometimes "game the clock"—improving the score without meaningfully changing lifespan.

Another problem is that mapping aging onto chronological time takes something nonlinear and maps it to a linear scale. But we know that the rate of aging is different during different periods of life. A 70-year-old accumulates more damage each year than a 30-year-old. This is because the older we get, the less effective our repair mechanisms become. Research has also found that adults typically go through accelerated periods of aging in their 40s and 60s. It might be more motivational to estimate the total damage and risk associated with a biological age score, rather than just thinking of it in terms of chronological age. One year of damage is more dangerous the older you are.

In addition to aging at different rates over time, your body also ages at different rates in different organs, tissues, and even cells. Organ aging rates can vary randomly, as well as by behavior, environment, and genetics. Someone who drinks alcohol might have a relatively old liver compared to the rest of their body, while someone who sunbathes might have relatively old skin. Someone with the inherited gene variant APOE4 might have a relatively old brain.

Some research groups are now moving to organ-specific clocks, which will be an improvement, but still hide important information. Do you have a 50-year-old heart because of cell population changes or protein aggregation? Not all types of damage are equally bad, nor will they respond the same way to different interventions. The single measures from biological clocks hide the underlying complexity of damage and give little information about the solutions needed to address it. Still, it's good to know something about the relative health of your organs, so these clocks are better than nothing.

Other groups are taking things further. They have found that even different parts of the same organ age at different rates. For example, when you look at the aging of different parts of the brain, you can see a correlation between the more aged areas and lower performance in whatever functions those areas govern. Understanding these variations can help prioritize technological development and treatment options for individuals.

While biological age tests are useful, and organ-level tests will be more useful, even these will eventually be superseded by tests that can provide actionable insights by detailing the amount of specific types of damage in each part of the body.

In the meantime, what can we do to keep our biological age below our chronological age? Damage is inevitable because of the nature of our biochemistry. No biological process can be perfectly efficient and, with the countless vibrating and interacting molecules that make up our bodies, little things go wrong all the time. However, even if damage is inevitable, aging isn't. Aging is reversible simply by reducing whatever damage has accumulated.

For example, an unhealthy lifestyle might lead to the early accumulation of damage that your body would repair if it had the chance. Smokers severely damage their lungs but, even after decades of abuse, quitting can give the body the breathing room it needs to heal.

Lifestyle can only take you so far, though, because some damage occurs just from being alive. Even so, your total burden of damage can go down dramatically if you turn your life around after years of late nights vaping, drinking, and eating candied bacon.

Lifestyle choices can cause large shifts in the level of accumulated damage. But there's no diet or exercise that can completely reverse even a single type of damage to zero, let alone all types of damage. Fortunately, your body's innate mechanisms aren't the only way to reverse aging. Drugs, gene therapies, and replacement therapies can fix damage, including types we can't heal on our own.

Key Takeaways

Historically, the medical industry has focused on treating diseases after they occur. Longevity technology, however, adopts a proactive approach. It seeks to intervene before diseases develop by targeting the aging process itself, the single biggest risk factor for most chronic diseases.

This shift in focus from treatment to prevention could revolutionize health care and lead to unprecedented improvements not just in your lifespan but also healthspan, which is the period of your life during which you're healthy. Modern medicine has done a good job extending lifespan, but not healthspan. People often spend their last years suffering. Radical life extension can't be achieved without increasing healthspan, and that will only be possible by focusing on the damage that's the root cause of age-related disease.

In other words, pursuing therapies that target age-related damage will not only keep people alive, but will also postpone chronic conditions. That way people can live not just longer, but also healthier lives.

Most people don't regard aging as a disease. However, if a disease is a condition that progressively degrades the performance of your body or mind, then aging qualifies. It's a special kind of disease, characterized by diverse and diffuse damage throughout the body that creates a positive feedback loop. The more damage you have, the more your systems are out of order, the less damage they can repair, and the more quickly you move away from a healthy state.

Aging leads to death by a thousand cuts, each causing minor dysfunction that's manageable at first but eventually wreaks havoc. Due to this diversity, we have useful models of aging, but it has not been fully characterized.

So, we can ask once again: what is aging? Aging is the process by which living organisms accumulate a variety of molecular damage throughout their bodies over their lifetimes. That damage comes from biological processes, random chance, and the environment. Damage is impossible to stop completely, but it can be slowed and it can be repaired.

The key thing to remember is that, while we don't know everything about the aging process, we know enough to develop the first generation of anti-aging technologies. These therapies won't be perfect but, if we choose the right approaches, they will have a real impact.

Choosing the right strategy isn't easy. There are potential ways to treat aging that won't work. Worse, there are many that will work, but the size of the effect will be so small that all the effort and excitement that go into them will be wasted. So it's important to be able to distinguish roads that lead to progress from detours and distractions.

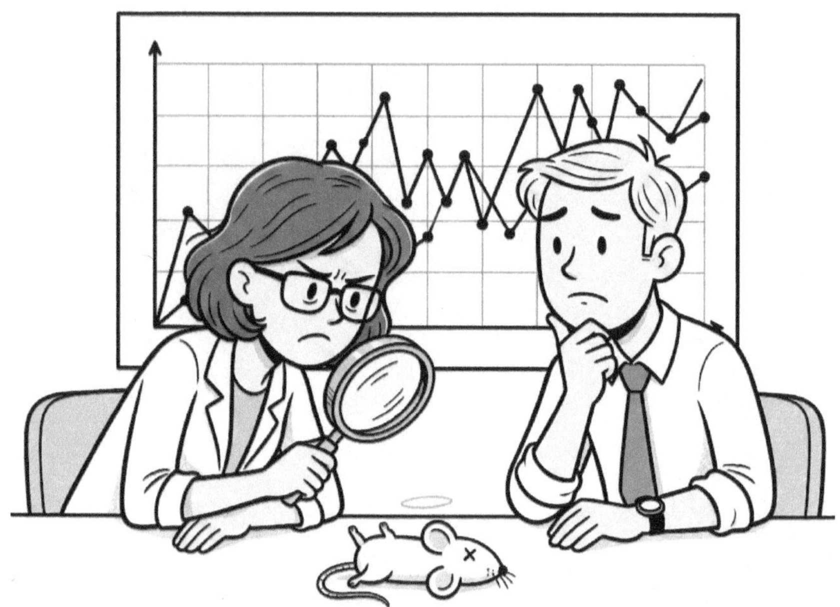

CHAPTER 3

DEAD ENDS

Every attempt to solve aging has failed. In hindsight, it's easy to see why. The failed attempts hinged on hypothetical singular "root causes" of aging, but as we've seen, aging isn't a single problem with a single solution. Instead, we now know that it's a multitude of processes that are individually deadly—solving just one aspect doesn't solve aging.

Yet the hope that a singular or simple solution to aging will be found is pernicious. While you don't need to fully understand aging to help bring about radical life extension, you do need to know enough to avoid seductive but counterproductive notions about longevity.

It's often painfully obvious whether a therapy has the potential to lead to radical life extension or would only lead to marginal benefit even in the best-case scenario. Spending too much time on marginal strategies is penny wise and pound foolish. Even if they produce something useful, the time and resources they consume could have gone to more critical-path research and technology development. Don't let yourself fall into the death trap of chasing small gains.

This is important, because the huge demand for longevity therapies has attracted a variety of people and opinions on how best to deal with the problem of aging. Many of these actors are selling snake oil—some unwittingly, others by pushing therapies with only marginal effects.

Regardless of their intentions, such products will make no meaningful difference in the end.

To make this less abstract, let's review what people have tried and why they were unsuccessful.

Calorie Restriction

One of the earliest strategies for life extension was calorie restriction. Calorie restriction means eating quite a bit less than normal while still getting adequate nutrients. Early studies, in which one group of rats ate normally and another was calorie restricted, showed that the restricted rats lived much longer. Subsequently, this was shown to extend lifespan for many types of animals, including rodents, canines, and nonhuman primates. The repeatability of these results was very exciting, and some people adopted restrictive diets to try to get similar health benefits.

Unfortunately, the potential of calorie restriction to extend human lifespan isn't obvious. One reason is that short-lived species have evolved responses to famines that work to get them to the next period of abundance. If you usually live for only two years, getting an extra six months is a huge 25% boost to lifespan. This might be the difference between reproducing and not reproducing. However, winters and droughts are less problematic for longer-lived species, which show considerably smaller lifespan gains when calorie restricted.

Even more disappointing was the realization in later studies that many of the animals used in these experiments overeat in lab conditions, so putting them on a diet simply prevents them from getting fat and unhealthy. In this case, it isn't calorie restriction that extends lifespan, but overeating that shortens it.

By contrast, mouse strains that naturally eat a healthy amount can be hurt by calorie restriction. Not only do these moderate-eaters receive no longevity boost from calorie restriction, but they actually die faster.

Most humans in modern society tend to overeat, so restricting calorie intake is likely to be a good idea for many people. Maintaining a healthy weight will help prevent you from dying prematurely. Humans may even live slightly longer on a severely restricted diet, but the effect appears to be marginal at best. So don't count on calorie counting to save you.

Antioxidants

A more recent strategy that got many people excited was the use of antioxidants. Oxidative damage occurs when your metabolism or your environment causes molecules in your body to become highly reactive. Examples include free radicals and charged molecules called reactive oxygen species that like to randomly steal electrons from other molecules in your body. This oxidizes the victim molecule and can cause it to stop working properly. A common example is oxidized cholesterol. Normal cholesterol helps keep your cell membranes strong and flexible, but oxidized cholesterol can weaken them and interfere with other biological processes that depend on healthy cell membranes. Similarly, oxidation can damage proteins and DNA.

The idea that oxidative damage was the root cause of aging became very popular in the 1980s. Given that assumption, people thought that if they took antioxidants it would help slow aging. It's true that your body needs antioxidants to help deal with reactive oxygen species that are produced as part of metabolic processes. It's also true that your body can absorb antioxidants from your diet.

However, when tested, antioxidant supplementation seemed to either not help or actually harm people. We eventually learned that reactive oxygen species are necessary signaling molecules, and having a large amount of antioxidants can disrupt important biological processes, like the benefits of exercise. That may be why, in spite of the huge volumes of antioxidant supplements being sold every year, this has not led to longer lives.

Telomeres

Another failed strategy was targeting telomeres. Telomeres are special sequences at the very end of your DNA strands that protect them from damage. Telomeres get shorter each time a cell divides. If they get short enough, cells can no longer divide and become dysfunctional. This contributes to cell depletion, inflammation, and other problems associated with aging.

When it was discovered in the 1980s that telomeres could be extended, people began to wonder if reversing telomere shortening could be a longevity therapy. Perhaps telomeres were like a ticking time bomb, causing key cell populations to decline until you drop dead. The natural experiment was to force the extension of telomeres to see if it could extend lifespan. It was tried in laboratory animals and, while it did seem to make mice a little healthier, it didn't cure aging or even rank as the most effective way to extend mouse lifespan.

Later we learned that telomere length isn't strongly associated with age in humans. Some old people have longer telomeres than young people. Extending telomeres can help with specific conditions, such as when someone has a rare genetic disease that causes accelerated telomere shortening. It can also help in specific tissues, but it won't do much to help with the aging of cells like neurons that don't divide. It also carries some serious risks. Finite telomere length protects an organism from cancer and, if you artificially lengthen telomeres, you can increase cancer risk. Artificially lengthening them can also have negative consequences for the immune system, tissue structure, and cell health.

Sirtuins

Another failed strategy was targeting sirtuin genes, which influence cellular gene expression patterns and genomic stability. These genes are involved in DNA repair, inflammation, metabolism, and mitochondrial function. In the 1990s it was shown that increasing sirtuin activity could extend lifespan in yeast, worms, and flies. Then, in the 2000s, it was discovered that a component of red wine called resveratrol could activate sirtuins and extend lifespan in various organisms.

People got excited about a natural compound that could potentially slow or reverse aging. Many companies started selling it as a supplement. Some companies developed drugs to mimic or enhance the effect, all in the hope that upregulating sirtuin activity would extend healthspan and lifespan in humans too.

Unfortunately, it doesn't. Later studies failed to replicate early results, and it was eventually discovered that poor experimental design in the original study had led to the misleading results. Resveratrol's reputation continued to unravel as it was revealed that it doesn't even activate sirtuins as initially claimed, let alone having the claimed benefits.

Despite this, many people are still buying resveratrol and analogs, even though there's no evidence it improves longevity. Later, people thought other compounds, like nicotinamide riboside, might upregulate sirtuins better, but they didn't meaningfully impact aging either. So, while sirtuins are an important part of human biology, they aren't a strong lever for longevity.

Repurposed Drugs

Another failed strategy that's still given too much attention is the use of rapamycin and other mTOR inhibitors—drugs that block mTOR, the cell's nutrient-sensing controller for growth and metabolism. Rapamycin mimics the effects of calorie restriction, so you can extend lifespan in laboratory animals without reducing their calorie intake. We would like to have our cake and eat it too, but unfortunately rapamycin doesn't seem to have the desired effect in humans. It also has potentially dangerous side effects like immune system suppression, toxicity, and metabolic dysregulation.

Another supposed wonder drug is metformin. This is a drug for diabetics that reduces blood sugar and seems to be helpful in treating diabetes. Tantalizing early results suggested that diabetics who took the drug had a lower incidence of cancer and other ailments. So the drug seemed to not only help with diabetes, but also help people live longer in general. However, when randomized clinical trials were run, no meaningful benefits were seen beyond its benefit to diabetics. So don't bet on metformin to add years to your life.

The list goes on. Single causes and cures of aging have repeatedly been hypothesized, tested, and falsified. This cycle will continue as we learn more about human biology and interventions are developed to treat different aspects of aging. A scientist will learn something about biology and a reporter will ask what big, exciting implications it has. The scientist will say, "Well, it's possible that it could help with aging," and so the clickbait headline will be, "Have scientists found a cure for aging?"

It is best to be skeptical of any proposed solution to aging, anything that supposedly reverses some aspect of aging, or even something that purportedly slows aging. It's a seriously hard problem to solve, and the solution won't be found at your local pharmacy.

Animal Experiments

Another rule of thumb is to be skeptical of any results that seem promising in animals. Many longevity strategies work in rodents but fail in humans. Examples include calorie restriction, reduced growth hormone, rapamycin, steroids, acarbose, methionine restriction, intermittent fasting, and metformin. Even in combination, these don't make mice live forever, and all of these interventions will have smaller effect sizes in humans than in mice. For example, calorie restriction can increase lifespan for some types of mice by 10-30%, but we would expect, at the very most, low single-digit percentage benefit for humans.

This is even more relevant for animals that are further removed from humans and have less in common biologically. Whereas calorie restriction can cause rats to live 30% longer, mice with one of their growth hormones downregulated can live 70% longer. Fruit flies that are calorie restricted, kept in a cold, dark box, and given mTOR inhibitors can live more than twice as long as their natural lifespans. That's nothing, since roundworms with mutations to their insulin and nutrient sensing genes can live five times as long. This is impressive until you hear from the mighty yeast, which says "hold my beer" while living 10 times as long when it's given two nutrient sensing mutations and calorie restriction.

These numbers are exciting until you realize that each step up the evolutionary ladder shrinks the effect: what works incredibly well in yeast works less well in worms, less well again in flies, and less well still in mice, with almost nothing carrying over cleanly to humans. That doesn't mean nothing will work in humans. It just means that tricks that dramatically extend the lives of simple organisms have much smaller impact on complex, long-lived species like us, so we will need more powerful approaches to extend human lifespan.

One of the problems with cross-species translatability of therapies is that different species age differently. Short-lived species tend to die quickly from things that long-lived species have evolved ways of dealing with. For example, mice are much more likely to die of cancer than elephants, despite the elephant having more cells and also a longer life over which mutations can occur. That's because elephants have developed more robust cancer suppression mechanisms, like extra copies of the p53 gene that codes for a tumor suppressor protein. Another is more stringent DNA damage detection during the cell cycle that more aggressively kills suspicious cells.

This is one of the reasons it's easier to extend life in short-lived animals than in long-lived ones. Short-lived species are lacking many simple things that could make them live longer, but didn't have the evolutionary pressure to develop or maintain them. Long-lived species, however, tend to already have solutions to many of the easy problems built into their biology, so only the difficult problems remain.

One way to think about this is that short-lived species have a relatively unstable biology, where their bodies have fewer feedback and repair mechanisms. This is an advantage in the wild because, instead of investing energy into longevity, they can develop and reproduce more quickly. Grow quickly into adulthood, reproduce, and then fall apart.

Humans don't do that. We live much longer than we need to reproduce. We even live longer than necessary to get our offspring to reproductive age. Our bodies are quite good at maintaining homeostasis. Even people who don't take good care of themselves can live much longer than most animals. With such a stable biological system, we enjoy longer lives. But we also have time to accumulate damage that's much more difficult to repair. For example, mice don't develop certain neurodegenerative diseases that are common in humans, because there isn't enough time in their lives to accumulate the plaques in their brains that would cause these problems.

So raise an incredulous eyebrow whenever experimental results in animals seem too good to be true.

How to Evaluate Strategies

With all of the noise and confusion around longevity, you need to be able to distinguish between fraudulent, marginal, and radical life extension. You don't need to fully understand the science, or be an expert in every area. You only need to develop an intuition for what people are trying to accomplish and a rough idea of the impact it will have. A fancy new drug that targets a circulating molecule that's strongly associated with age might sound promising, but how excited should you be? Should you invest your energy or resources into it, or are your efforts better spent elsewhere? Carefully choosing how to allocate your time and money is critical. There are many roads to walk down, but most of them are dead ends—both figuratively and literally.

One rule of thumb is to gauge how a proposed therapy compares to diet and exercise. A healthy lifestyle won't radically extend your lifespan, but it has the potential to add many years to your life. When someone proposes the development of some new therapy, one question to ask is whether the proposed effect size is measured in decades, years, or months. If you get only a 1% gain in lifespan, you would need 10 such therapies to achieve the results you get from going for a run every day—and that's assuming the effects are additive, which isn't generally the case. A therapy is more likely to be meaningful if it can improve health as much as regular exercise. If it can't, then it probably isn't something that should get a lot of time or attention.

For example, you could probably improve your health a little by periodically eating a diet very low in methionine—an essential amino acid that, when restricted, triggers more cellular recycling and some of the effects seen with calorie restriction. So should we create companies to provide methionine-restricted meals? You might make a profit, but for the average person the effect is smaller than a healthy diet or exercise, so it doesn't pass the bar of an exciting strategy. Worse, such meals promote a false sense of security and divert time and resources from technologies with far higher potential value.

Another litmus test is to consider whether a proposed therapy should be taken by all older, but otherwise healthy, adults. If a treatment really targets aging, then it should be helpful to everyone. If someone proposes the development of a drug or technology that only helps in a very specific case, then it's unlikely that it will lead to radical life extension. This is true even if it treats some symptoms of aging, because treating some effects of aging won't greatly impact how long you live.

Using older but otherwise healthy adults as a criterion is important because we don't want to chase problems that stem from common lifestyle choices, like smoking, drinking alcohol, or overeating. Mitigating the effects of an unhealthy lifestyle is a laudable goal, but it will divert resources from solving the more fundamental and universal problems of aging. The potential impact of a drug that cures alcohol-induced liver disease may be large, but it's tiny compared to the impact of a therapy that treats liver aging. So the same resources might save one person from dying of hepatitis or hundreds of people from dying of age-related disease. Work that targets age-related damage will tend to solve more conditions, save more people, and make a greater contribution to radical life extension.

Another way to classify different therapies is by whether they attempt to slow aging or reverse aging. Either could make you live longer and delay age-related disease, but slowing aging would primarily benefit the young, while reversing aging could help everyone.

Another important consideration is whether a strategy can affect the entire body, or just a portion of it. Many companies sell beauty products that claim to keep skin looking young and healthy but, even if those worked, your internal organs and tissues would continue to age. Aging is a body-wide process that needs to be handled comprehensively as it only takes one weak link to kill you. If a therapy is too narrow, or has no chance of working more broadly, then it's less appealing and should get correspondingly less attention.

For any particular proposal, you should also consider what the side effects would be. A cure for aging that left you permanently bald would be tolerable. But a drug that might only slightly increase lifespan, while putting you at risk of serious debilitation or illness, would not. The smaller the benefit, the less tolerable even moderate risks become. This is because you would need to combine many small-effect therapies for radical life extension, but the side effects would also combine in nasty ways. The risk of drug interactions or unintended consequences will grow, capping both the number of such therapies you could take and their potential benefit.

A typical drug has what is called a therapeutic window. If you don't take enough, then you don't get benefits. If you take too much, you get sick or maybe even die. The difference between the minimum amount for benefit and the maximum amount before serious side effects is the therapeutic window. This is easy enough to manage for one drug, but if you take more than one, they can interact and interfere with each other. You might need more of one, or it might no longer be safe to take as much of another. These complex interactions can make it difficult or impossible to find safe and effective doses for large numbers of drugs in combination.

Drug development for radical life extension is hard because human biology is extremely complex. Each cell contains hundreds of thousands of distinct molecules, most still uncataloged and many taking on multiple roles, so a drug that helps one symptom can easily break something elsewhere. That's why so many drugs fail in clinical trials: they seem to work at first, but side effects make them too dangerous. We can't even cure simple diseases—statins, the most popular drugs of all time, can't reliably halt the progression of atherosclerosis, the buildup of fatty plaque in your arteries, let alone reverse it.

Another trap is becoming enamored with elegant but inefficient solutions. One example is the allotopic expression of mitochondrial DNA, which just means moving mitochondrial genes into the cell nucleus and modifying them so that the proteins they produce are transported into the mitochondria. Mitochondria have their own DNA, and it gets rather beaten up over time because of the reactive molecules that are generated as mitochondria produce the energy-storing molecules called ATP. As mitochondrial DNA gets damaged, it causes the mitochondria to misbehave, producing less energy and causing the cells to be less effective at their jobs. If mitochondrial DNA is the vending machine at your office that sometimes goes out of order, then allotopic expression is food delivery.

Some mitochondrial genes are already stored in the cell nucleus, and those are relatively well protected from damage compared to the ones that reside inside mitochondria. So it makes sense that you could improve the situation by moving the rest there as well. Unfortunately, this is a hard thing to do, so hard that evolution has not come up with a solution over billions of years.

So even though allotopic expression of mitochondrial DNA would be better and some proof of concept work has led to early successes, we must bear in mind that the time and money going into this approach has opportunity costs. Choosing the wrong opportunities means that the people right on the edge, who would have survived if longevity technology arrived sooner, won't.

To pursue radical life extension effectively, we need a very specific kind of skepticism. Be wary of interventions that have already proved to be dead ends, no matter how hyped they are. Treat results that exist only in experimental animals—especially evolutionarily distant ones— as weak evidence. Be cautious of therapies with tiny effect sizes, that only affect a narrow part of the body, or that only address a single disease. Likewise, be doubtful about small-molecule approaches: they tend to have small benefits and broad side effects, and they generally act at the level of human metabolism rather than directly removing damage. And be skeptical of strategies that merely slow the accumulation of damage instead of reversing it; slowing can be worth pursuing when repair is too hard or there's genuine low-hanging fruit, but only if the effect size justifies the opportunity cost.

Evaluating Ongoing Efforts

While there are many strategies for longevity, from the perspective of radical life extension most of them are dead in the water. This may seem to imply a negative outlook. Nothing works, and the world is full of scams. There's some truth to that. Nonetheless, new technologies continue to be proposed and some look promising for real rejuvenation.

Even though new technologies are exciting, we should assess them dispassionately so we keep realistic expectations. Otherwise, it's easy to fall into a different trap: becoming enamored of partial solutions. We want to use the latest tools and technology without slipping into wishful thinking, so we should never assume that any single technique will solve a complex problem like aging on its own. Longevity has already gone through many cycles of discovery and hype, so it's worth naming some of the latest examples so you can see which tools might help, but only as small pieces of a larger puzzle.

First, let's look at stem cell therapy. Stem cells are the body's source of fresh replacement cells, and the therapy involves having a doctor inject specific types of cells into your body with the hope that they will rejuvenate you. In very specific cases, like bone marrow failure and leukemias, stem cell transplantation has led to high cure rates. However, as a general approach to treating aging, stem cell injections are less impressive. They appear to help to some extent, but the underlying mechanisms are unclear. It seems likely that most of the benefit from general purpose stem cell therapies comes from the signaling molecules that the cells release, which improve the microenvironment for the rest of the cells in your body.

Stem cells are important to maintaining a healthy body and are lost as we age. But getting stem cell injections typically doesn't produce a lasting benefit. Even as cell replacement therapy becomes better and these cells are able to get to the right locations and engraft properly, there are types of damage that stem cells won't be able to solve. In particular, new cells will be unable to fully repair the extracellular matrix. The ECM is also a problem for cell therapy because damaged ECM prevents cells from behaving correctly, so the expected benefit from new cells could decrease over time as the ECM degrades. That said, future versions of cell therapies probably will be part of the toolkit that helps people live radically longer lives.

Next, we can look at senolytics, which are drugs that clear senescent cells. Cellular senescence occurs when cells enter a state of cell cycle arrest. They stop dividing and also send out signals that are used in wound repair. Your immune system then goes and clears them out. As you get old, your immune system can no longer remove them as quickly as they are produced, so they accumulate and cause chronic inflammation and other problems.

Fortunately, you can kill senescent cells by taking senolytic compounds. Killing senescent cells has been shown to partially rejuvenate mice, but the effect on humans is still unknown. Clearing senescent cells isn't a full solution to aging, because it doesn't address other types of age-related damage, like cancer. We don't yet know how well this strategy will work, but many companies are now developing senolytic therapies, and it may become a useful tool to fight aging.

Next, partial reprogramming. Partial reprogramming is a relatively new development, whereby cells can be given chemical signals that restore their gene expression patterns to a more youthful state. This improves the way the cell performs its duties and helps it act like a younger cell. The promise of partial reprogramming is that it could extend both healthspan and lifespan by improving organ and tissue function. This would be accomplished by improving the effectiveness of cells in each tissue or organ, as well as the cells of the immune system and the stem cells that produce somatic cells—the ordinary working cells that make up your tissues.

A lot of money has been poured into partial reprogramming, and hopefully it will generate some useful therapies for extending healthspan and lifespan. Unfortunately, the best it can do is help the body clear out damage that it already knows how to remove, with no ability to reverse other kinds of damage. For example, partial reprogramming won't be able to reverse DNA mutations. So it won't solve aging on its own, but it could potentially be a useful therapy.

Finally, let's consider artificial intelligence. AI is a tool that can help us understand human biology and aging, and assist with drug development, gene therapies, surgical protocols, and more. It's therefore a real boon for longevity and will help us move faster toward curing aging. However, it isn't yet sufficient to solve any of the root causes of aging, and may not be for decades. This isn't because AI won't be smart enough, but because AI won't have sufficient data. Without large, high-quality datasets, AI struggles to produce useful insights. For example, AI only cracked the protein-folding problem after decades of work by scientists and volunteers to map the 3D structures of proteins. In general, generating the right kinds of data for AI to analyze is an ongoing project that could take a long time and a lot of money.

This data collection would not matter as much if we could use computers to emulate cells, but the computational power for a predictive, high-fidelity emulation of a human cell at the atomic level remains a profound challenge. This doesn't mean that progress can't be made in the interim. It only means that we should not expect or depend on a sudden breakthrough from artificial intelligence that will make all other efforts to solve aging irrelevant. An AI-derived solution to aging needs a lot of time and attention and won't simply happen on its own.

Using AI to accelerate our understanding and potential manipulation of human biology makes sense, but the problem is still enormous. It's difficult not only to manipulate human biology, but even to understand it. Physicists have a pretty good handle on atoms and stars, but biologists have not yet fully mapped the functional interactions and precise concentrations of the molecules that make up the human body. If solving aging with AI requires us to first fully datamine human biology, there's little hope that it will lead to radical life extension in our lifetimes.

Almost unlimited resources could be poured into scientific research into how the human body works on the cellular and organismal level. If we did that, we would be in a much better position to develop drugs that manipulate human metabolism. Yet, if we spend all our time learning, we won't spend any time developing therapies that could save lives in the meantime and many people will die unnecessarily as a result.

Key Takeaways

There have been many failed strategies for treating aging, either because they don't help, or because their effect size is too small. So reflect on these failures to learn from them and gain the wisdom to do better. If something sounds too good to be true, it probably is. If it isn't clear that a therapy could make a difference, it probably won't.

There are technologies in development that could help, but not enough resources to pursue them all. Time is of the essence, and we should be heavily biased toward solutions that can have a large impact quickly, even if there are alternatives that would have other advantages. People are dying every day, and what people decide to do impacts when the bloodbath will end.

Sadly, most people who pursue longevity never realize this and spend their time working on low-impact projects. There are thousands of scientists hacking at the branches of aging for every researcher who is striking at the root. They may get fame or fortune, but they don't make a dent in the problem of death.

If you want to be sure your own efforts are going toward effective solutions for radical life extension, you will need a basic understanding of what you are and how aging kills you.

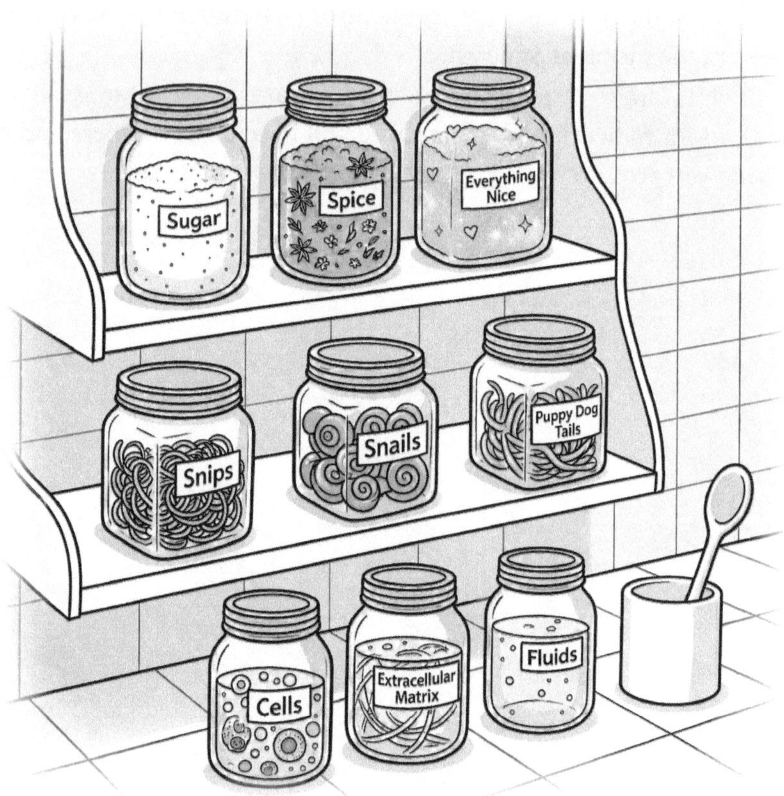

Sugar
Spice
Everything Nice
Snips
Snails
Puppy Dog Tails
Cells
Extracellular Matrix
Fluids

CHAPTER 4

CELLS, EXTRACELLULAR MATRIX, AND FLUIDS

Nobody completely understands how the human body works. You might be able to name every bone in the skeleton, but you won't find anyone who can tell you what every cell type or molecule does. If solving aging required a complete understanding of human biology, our prognosis would be poor. Fortunately, developing longevity technology only requires a working knowledge of how a healthy body functions and how aging causes dysfunction. What follows is a brief introduction to those topics from the perspective of someone who wants to bring about radical life extension. Think of it as the minimum theory you need to lay the foundation and get started—enough to orient you in the field, but not enough to get you into medical school.

The goal here is to give you a sense of which topics and ideas matter most for longevity technology. If you don't have a background in biology, you should read *Molecular Biology of the Cell* by Bruce Alberts. It will give you enough knowledge of biology to understand the specific problems of aging and the solutions being proposed. It will also help you absorb more advanced information from specialized books and papers, and participate in discussions on longevity topics, making you more effective. Also, molecular biology is beautiful to behold, so hike up that mountain of knowledge and enjoy the view.

It won't stop there, though. You'll need to keep learning, because advances are being made every day. The flood of information can be overwhelming, so you'll quickly need to distinguish what is important to longevity, what is merely nice to know, and what is totally irrelevant. News sources, even ones dedicated to longevity, often publish articles that boil down to "exercise is good for you." Learning to ignore that kind of unhelpful content will save you precious time and make it easier to spot the hidden gems, like reports of new technologies that could become therapies or experiments that reveal useful clues about aging damage.

What Are You?

In the meantime, let's start with some basics. The goal is to keep you alive, but what are you? Not your genes, not your body, but something in your brain. Not the whole brain, but the defining parts of your personality, memories, preferences, and so on. Everything else is just a support system that keeps you alive and allows you to interact with the world. If you cut your hair, you're still you. The same goes if you lose an arm, a leg, or a kidney. The point is that, in human biology, not all parts of your body are equally important. The most important thing to protect is the brain.

Human biology reflects this with the blood-brain barrier. Your brain has a protective layer of cells that sits between it and the blood vessels that flow through it. Just as your skin helps keep your body safe from pathogens, the blood-brain barrier is an extra layer of defense for your brain.

The brain has many neurons, but also large numbers of helper cells. The most common are oligodendrocytes, which act as electrical insulation for neurons. Astrocytes maintain a healthy environment for neurons and microglia are the brain's immune cells. Among others, these brain cells form structures that keep your heart beating, regulate temperature, and allow you to think and feel.

It's currently possible to keep a brain alive outside the body by putting it in a jar and supplying it with blood. For example, pig brains have been kept alive outside of the body for hours under specialized perfusion systems. However, this doesn't work for very long because the body does a lot of work to keep the brain alive, and we don't yet have the technology to replicate all of it. For now, keeping you alive means keeping both your brain and the rest of your body healthy.

Most people would say that the human body is made up of cells, but they would only be half right. Half your body is your cells and half is a combination of extracellular matrix, bodily fluids, bacteria, and other things. You actually have roughly as many bacterial cells in your body as human cells. The bacteria are much smaller, live mainly in your intestines, and only add a couple hundred grams of mass.

The second biggest component of your body is the extracellular matrix, or ECM. The ECM is structural scaffolding that your cells produce to make your bones rigid, your joints flexible, and your skin soft. The overall shape of your body and its internal structure is determined by where cells lay down ECM. Within that ECM, your 30 trillion cells do their various jobs to keep you alive.

ECM is specialized to specific tissues. The ECM around neurons is soft, like a leather armchair that a professor uses to sit and think. The ECM of bones is strong, like the wood a carpenter uses to make a house. If you took the wood out of a tree, its bark and leaves would fall into a pile on the ground. Similarly, if you took away a person's ECM, they would collapse into a puddle of cells and bodily fluids. It's hard to be a multicellular organism without ECM.

The third major component of your body is fluids. Your bodily fluids aren't just water, but complex soups of proteins, sugars, fats, and other molecular structures. Blood is one such fluid, but there are others, including cerebrospinal fluid, which nurtures your central nervous system; interstitial fluid, which surrounds cells in tissues; the humors in your eyes; and lymph, which drains from your tissues back to your bloodstream. These fluids keep your cells and tissues clean, deliver nutrients and remove wastes, and carry signaling molecules that affect cell and organ behavior. For example, when you eat, your bloodstream fills with insulin; this signal tells cells it's time for them to eat as well, by absorbing glucose from your blood plasma.

You wouldn't survive without your fluids. When a plant is unable to get enough water, it shrivels into a stiff shadow of its former glory.

Similarly, if you took away a person's fluids they would be like a mummy: a human-shaped piece of beef jerky.

On the other hand, if you took away a person's cells, they would basically be a big, wet sponge with some bones inside. It takes cells, ECM, and fluids to make a person and, with all three, you're an incredible piece of machinery.

At least, you are when you're young. As you get older, all three parts start to have problems. Your cells stop performing their jobs or, worse, do things that are actively detrimental. Your ECM starts to get hard where it should be soft, soft where it should be hard, full of holes where it should be solid, and impermeable where it should allow fluid to flow. And your fluids get filled with junk and inflammatory factors that cause your cells and ECM to malfunction.

Experiments with older animals have shown that restoring cells, ECM, or fluids to a more youthful state can make the animal healthier and help it live longer. Conversely, old cells, ECM, or fluids can make a young animal unhealthy and lead to an early death. So a lot of the work of longevity technology is to restore cells, ECM, and bodily fluids to a youthful state. To be effective in that endeavor, you need to understand how damage accumulates in and affects each of them.

Cells

When people are first taught about cells, they are told they are little balls of fluid with a nucleus and some other organelles: like a water balloon with a few marbles floating around inside. In reality, they are more like little transformer robots that can change their shape and composition to do different things.

The interior of the cell contains a fluid called cytoplasm but, just as your bodily fluids are full of cells and other molecules, that fluid is jam-packed with organelles and molecules like proteins and nucleic acids. So picture a water balloon with Lego pieces crowding the interior and covering the outside. The largest structure inside is the nucleus, a sphere that contains the cell's DNA. Proteins in the nucleus read the DNA to produce RNA, which is then shipped out so that other proteins can use it to build more proteins. Using DNA to create RNA is called transcription, because there's a one-to-one match between segments of DNA and segments of RNA. Using RNA to make proteins is called translation: three RNA nucleotides are used to select which amino acid to add to a growing protein chain. For example, 30 nucleotides of RNA would map to 10 amino acids along a protein. The mapping from nucleotides to amino acids is called the genetic code.

While DNA and RNA are composed of only 4 types of nucleotides, proteins are made from 20 different types of segments called amino acids. The translation process picks which of the amino acids should be next in the protein. Each amino acid has different properties it can contribute to a protein, adding strength, flexibility, electrostatic charge, chemically reactive sites, and so on. This is part of what makes proteins so useful; the amino acids that compose them have a wider range of chemical properties than nucleotides. This, and the fact that they are smaller, allows them to fold themselves into more powerful machines than could be made with just RNA.

When a protein is produced, it's a long strand. It then naturally folds up into a 3D shape which allows it to perform different functions. It might fold up into a pair of molecular scissors and cut other proteins. Or it might become a molecular clamp that pushes two molecules

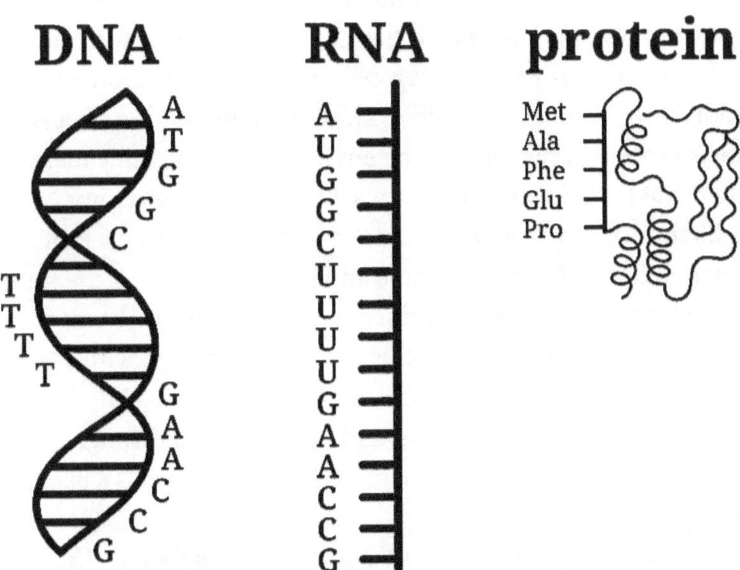

DNA is transcribed to RNA, which is sometimes translated to proteins.

together to combine them. Proteins can do many incredible things, all starting with a long chain of amino acids that folds up into a little machine. Notably, many RNAs aren't used for creating proteins and instead become little machines of their own.

The army of RNAs and proteins in a cell work together to help the cell control its shape, move around, ingest and expel molecules, and collaborate with other cells. Some proteins float around inside a cell, while others are embedded in the cell's outer membrane, its organelles, or vesicles secreted by the cells into the fluid around them. Sometimes multiple proteins will combine into a larger, more powerful protein complex, like when TV-show robots combine to form Voltron or Megazords.

There's a lot going on inside and on the surface of a cell, so a more accurate description requires a few details. First, the membrane that contains the cell is built on a lipid bilayer that would normally be pretty smooth. Cartoons of cells typically show a mostly bare surface where a few proteins anchor themselves. In truth, almost half of the cell membrane is composed of proteins that allow the cell to sense and interact with the outside world. The cell will look almost entirely covered in proteins because they anchor into the cell membrane like tree trunks, with much of each protein protruding to the outside or inside of the cell like the top of a tree. Just as it is hard to see the ground when flying above a dense forest, if you look at a cell from the outside, only a tiny fraction of the lipid bilayer is visible. These proteins are the means by which cells sense and respond to the environment, how they identify each other, and how they protect themselves like a suit of armor.

A cell's surface continuously changes as the cell makes new proteins that are shipped to the cell membrane and installed there. At the same time, the cell also sucks in parts of the membrane to ingest things from the environment in a process called endocytosis. The cell will also do the reverse and spit out molecules to do work or send signals. Meanwhile, molecules are flowing in and out of the cell through pores in the membrane, for example ion channels. The cell surface is a bustling and busy place.

The cell surface is dynamic in another way as well. The cell membrane is supported by a rigid structure called the cytoskeleton, which is like the rods that hold up a tent. Unlike a tent, the cytoskeleton can change shape, which allows cells to reach for things, move around, or even grow projections up to several meters long, like nerves do. By changing their shape, cells can engage in a wide range of complex behaviors, such as chasing bacteria, moving through various tissues in your body, and even engulfing and eating other cells.

If the cell surface sounds complex, it's nothing compared to what is going on inside the cell. The cytoplasm is the water-filled interior, but a cell isn't like a snow globe mostly filled with water with some little beads swirling around. It's jam-packed with structures, such as the endoplasmic reticulum, an organelle where proteins are synthesized, and mitochondria, which are like little power plants. These two types of structures, along with the nucleus, take up a third of the interior volume. Blueprints, factories, and power generators.

Another 15% is taken up by free-floating proteins, RNA, and other molecules. These are largely enzymes for speeding up chemical reactions, energy carriers, and signaling molecules. Workers, batteries, and communications networks.

Another 10% is occupied by smaller organelles like the Golgi apparatus and lysosomes, as well as the cytoskeleton. The Golgi apparatus ships proteins to various destinations while lysosomes break down old or damaged molecules to make parts for new ones, effectively recycling them. The cytoskeleton not only gives the cell structural support, but also provides an internal network of tubes and cords that are used as a transportation network.

This leaves a measly 40% of the space in the cell for regular old water. To visualize how dense and crowded a cell is, picture a bathtub that's filled 40% with water balloons of various sizes. Then you dump in buckets full of string, twigs, wind-up toys, rice, and other stuff until it's 60% filled. Finally, pour in water until the tub is full and you'll see a mess that somewhat approximates a cell.

And that's how life works. A cell is a small, isolated space where RNA and proteins make more of themselves using DNA, make or modify lipids and sugars, pull in energy, excrete waste, and occasionally copy DNA and split into two cells.

All these interactions between DNA, RNA, proteins, and other molecules influence each other in complex ways. For example, a certain type of RNA might cause a specific protein to be made, but then that protein might inhibit the production of that RNA. Such a feedback loop would be one small part of the genetic programs that control the behavior of the cell. Human cells have over 50,000 genes that can be used to make RNAs, so the number of potential interactions and feedback loops is enormous.

Things get even more complicated when you realize that these internal pathways are only part of the picture. Cells receive chemical signals from their environment and from other cells that impact their behavior. For example, this external control is how immune cells clean up viral infections. When they touch a cell and realize it's infected, they send a signal that tells the infected cell to kill itself.

Even if you have a perfectly healthy cell, it can go totally haywire if it gets the wrong external cues. Signals might come from the extracellular matrix via mechanical transduction, or neighboring cells via short-ranged signals called paracrine factors, or from distant cells via hormones. Cells are also affected by what you eat, and environmental factors like light and air particulates.

There are regulatory systems inside cells, outside of cells, and between cells. When all of them are working well, the cells and the organism are able to flourish. When they are disrupted, function and quality of life suffer. For example, if insulin signaling is disrupted, your cells stop taking up glucose which can lead to diabetes.

All of these processes and interactions can be thought of as biological computer programs or biological circuits. The program that's being run and the inputs determine what a cell does. It isn't totally arbitrary—cells tend to fall into specific roles called "cell types" like skin cells or liver cells through the process of cell differentiation, which is where a cell commits to performing a certain type of work.

In this way at least, cells are like people: they are all made of the same stuff, but they look different and have different jobs. If you have two children, one might become a lawyer and the other might become a doctor. Similarly, your cells split and take on different roles like kidney cells, fat cells, and so on. Changing a cell's job, or its cell type, requires it to physically transform. A liver cell looks very different from a neuron because its job requires a different shape, different proteins, and so on.

Though cells can change jobs, it's uncommon. Neurons don't normally turn into muscle cells and vice versa. The main thing controlling a cell's job is what genes are expressed in the cell. Gene expression is partly controlled by epigenetics, which are chemical modifications that don't change the DNA sequence, but alter whether genes are transcribed. If DNA is a piano, then epigenetics is the sheet music. Scientists can change a cell from one type to another by adjusting these DNA markers, which tell the cell to run a different program. Every cell has the same DNA, but heart cells and brain cells dance to a different tune.

There are hundreds of different cell types, all with the same DNA but running different genetic programs. These differences lead to a wide range of cell shapes and behaviors. Nerve cells stretch out to build communication lines. A red blood cell is good at transporting oxygen and passively slipping through capillaries, while a white blood cell might be good at actively moving through different tissues to hunt down pathogens.

Some cells produce barriers to keep water and nutrients in, while keeping pathogens out. Some digest food. Some send signals throughout the body to orchestrate and coordinate different cells and tissues. Cells are continuously recycling molecules internally to change themselves, externally to adjust the mechanical properties of ECM, and many cell types do things that we don't yet understand.

A subset of cells have the important job of producing more cells. These are called stem cells, and when they divide they usually split into another stem cell and a somatic cell. The somatic cell then goes and does whatever job it has been assigned. Cells are dying all the time in your body, about 1% each day. You need stem cells to replenish the cells that are lost, or you will lose tissue mass and function. The rates differ depending on cell type; neurons are rarely replenished but also die less frequently. Other cells, such as the lining of your intestines, are replaced every week. Common types of cells by count are red blood cells, platelets, and skin cells. By mass, muscle cells usually dominate, followed by fat and liver cells.

Cellular Damage

With so many different types of cells, it may be no surprise that there is also a wide variety of ways cells go wrong with age. Many different factors can cause cells to misbehave. They might have internal damage, or they might be reacting to external stimuli in the ECM or in fluids. Or they might get direct signals from cell contact that cause them to do things that are counterproductive.

One problem shared across all cell types is maintaining a healthy number of cells of each type. If you don't have enough of certain cells, you will suffer from conditions like anemia, excess bleeding, skin atrophy, muscle wasting, metabolic disorders, and jaundice.

Things often go the other way, and that is why cancer is one of the top causes of death. Human cells are programmed to die unless they are told to stay alive by external signals. They are also programmed to die if they receive specific external signals to do so. So the body has mechanisms for limiting the number of cells. If cells stop obeying these rules, they can keep dividing out of control. This causes further damage, as the rapidly replicating cells physically encroach on and disrupt the function of surrounding healthy tissue, and eventually spread to distant parts of the body via metastasis.

Other behavioral switches occur with immune cells. The immune system is divided into the innate immune system and the adaptive immune system. Innate immune cells float around and respond to anything that looks like a typical pathogen or infection. For example, macrophages will eat bacteria, dying human cells, or other debris. They can switch between attack mode and repair mode; as you get older, they spend more time in attack mode, sometimes causing more harm than good. Similarly, neutrophils will eat pathogens, but they can also shoot out molecular nets to try to fight invaders. Natural killer cells will kill your own cells if they look like they are infected. All of these innate immune cells become less effective and more inflammatory as you get older.

The adaptive immune system targets specific pathogens. After the innate immune system kills some pathogens, some of the pieces will be shown to B cells and T cells from the adaptive immune system. These cells will then be prepared for the next time that specific pathogen shows up. During the next infection, the B cells will pump out antibodies that disable and flag the pathogen, making it easier to find and destroy. The T cells will quickly divide into a big army that hunts down cells infected by that specific pathogen, and then reduce their numbers greatly once the fight is over.

The adaptive immune system also adopts problematic behaviors with age. It's less able to learn to fight new pathogens. It also becomes less able to properly recognize your own body components and can start to fight against them; this is what autoimmune reactions are.

Cellular malfunction has many underlying causes, but some cellular processes are more critical than others. The most important are core functions like transcription, translation, and cell division. Genetic defects in these can disable critical processes and even prevent an organism from developing. Unsurprisingly, age-related damage that disrupts these can cause serious issues for adults. For example, as you get older your cells have a harder time producing long RNA strands. This biases the populations of RNAs and proteins toward shorter ones, negatively impacting cell function.

One type of damage in cells that's very difficult to repair is DNA mutations. Mutations are a special type of damage because DNA stores information. If the DNA breaks and is repaired incorrectly, it might be chemically normal with no oxidation or cross-links. Nevertheless, if the nucleotide sequence changes, it can change the genetic program that your cell is running, and the types of RNAs and proteins that are produced—dramatically affecting cell behavior.

DNA is also problematic because it's unique to a cell and only replicated when cells divide. So, whereas damage to other types of molecules can usually be mitigated by the production of new molecules, this turnover doesn't help in the case of DNA. A DNA mutation isn't always a problem, because sometimes it occurs in a somatic cell like a skin cell that's going to die soon anyway. And even in that skin cell, mutations usually don't interfere with the production of RNAs and proteins.

However, every once in a while, a mutation can occur in a stem cell. As that stem cell produces more and more daughter cells, the mutation is also replicated. This is called somatic mosaicism, where you get sub-populations of cells with slightly different DNA. Sometimes the mutations give the sub-population a growth advantage, and it spreads throughout a tissue. This is called clonal expansion, and a common example is age spots on the skin of older adults.

Age spots can be annoying, but the same process can be seriously life-threatening in other tissues. If similar mutations occur in your bone marrow, it can lead to problems like clonal hematopoiesis of indeterminate potential, which is where mutant cells take over large portions of your bone marrow and put you at greater risk of diseases like cancer.

A similar process can occur with mitochondria within a cell. If a mitochondrion's DNA is damaged, it might prevent it from working. For one mitochondrion of hundreds, this isn't such a problem, and bad mitochondria will eventually be recycled. However, certain mutations can have a proliferative effect. Just as bad cells can spread through clonal expansion, so too can bad mitochondria spread and take over the cell. This can cause the cell to go into a low-power state where it doesn't work as well. Poorly performing mitochondria can be a big problem for energy-hungry tissue like muscles and the brain.

Even without DNA mutations, gene expression suffers if damage occurs to the epigenetic control mechanisms in a cell. These are like on/off switches for genes and, as we age, more and more of them are accidentally switched in the wrong direction. It's like trying to fly a plane full of cats who like to jump on the control panel and swat the buttons. These random changes are called epigenetic drift, and make it hard for a cell to do its job.

Another type of damage is persistent viral infection. We all get viral infections during our lives, and many are cleared quickly, but some of these viruses hide inside our cells for years or decades. For example, most people in the world have herpes simplex virus-1 in their body, and almost everybody has varicella-zoster virus, which causes chickenpox and shingles. The symptoms may go away, but the virus is still in there. The virus in your body is damage, and the accumulation of persistent viruses is a type of aging. Moreover, these viruses cause progressively more damage as the immune system declines with age. For example, cytomegalovirus can lead to the persistent inflammation called inflammaging, which then confuses your immune system and makes it less effective.

Viruses hide in several ways. Sometimes they just create RNA that hangs out in a cell's cytoplasm, protected by special proteins. Some can hide their DNA in a cell nucleus. Certain types of viruses, such as HIV, can go even further, and incorporate their genetic information into your cell's DNA. If viral DNA gets into your germline cells before you have kids, then they might inherit it, too. Something like this has happened many times in the past: nearly half your genome is made of ancient mobile DNA, including about 8% that clearly comes from retroviruses that infected our ancestors.

The remnants of this ancient viral DNA can still be quite dangerous. For example, transposable elements are genes that instruct the cell to make additional copies of themselves or move to different places within the genome. The process looks like a viral attack, so it causes inflammation and can lead to autoimmune reactions. Not only that, but new insertions can destroy other genes in the process. Broken genes can degrade cell function and also lead to cancer. In youth, your body suppresses these transposable elements with epigenetic markers. However, as you age, damage to your epigenome releases these jumping genes to cause mayhem.

Human cells aren't the only ones that go from helpful to harmful as we age. The other half of your cells are little bacteria and other microbes inside your gut. Like a farmer, our immune system maintains a healthy population of microbes that digest the fiber we eat and produce helpful nutrients for us in a symbiotic relationship. As you get older, the gut population shifts from helpful microbes to harmful ones. An example of bad bacteria is Helicobacter pylori, which infects the stomach linings of almost half the people in the world. Bad bacteria can crowd out useful microbes, provoke immune reactions, get into your bloodstream, and cause other problems for your body. Just as there's damage when human cell populations shift from normal to cancerous, there's also damage when the gut microbiota shift from helpful to harmful. Microbes can also produce biofilms that make it harder for the body to clear them out, make them resistant to antibiotics, and disrupt normal body functions like wound healing.

There's much more to know about how cells work and how they break with age. For now, let's focus on another important, highly variable, dynamic, and occasionally problematic part of your body: the extracellular matrix. If you want to understand biology and aging deeply enough to be able to do something about it, you need to understand the ECM.

Extracellular Matrix

Your body is made of cells, but it also has other things like hair, tooth enamel, fingernails, lenses in your eyes, and bone. Recall that these and other noncellular components of your body are the extracellular matrix and, if cells are bees, then ECM is the beehive.

ECM is a specialized structure secreted by cells that they can attach themselves to. It gives them a place to live, or to grab when moving around. It's what allows cells to form the functional shapes of tissues and organs. ECM can be hard, like your teeth and bones. ECM can also be soft, as in the cartilage in your ears, or the elastic sacs of your lungs.

ECM is a nice place for your cells to live, but it also holds your body together and helps your cells cooperate to do things that they could not do on their own. For example, the cornea of your eye is mostly made of specialized ECM that has the right shape and transparency to focus light.

The most important function of ECM is to help cells stick together, so you can be the multicellular organism you were meant to be. The second most important function is providing barriers around different parts of your body. For example, your skin cells sit on top of a layer of extracellular matrix called the basement membrane, which supports them, provides signals, and serves as a fence to keep bad things out and good things in. ECM is also used to give shape and structure to the various organs and organ systems in your body.

These organs and tissues are constructed to suit the needs of different cell types, so the ECM that heart cells make is quite different from the ECM that brain cells build. Just like how a chef can make better food in a professional kitchen, your cells perform their jobs better when they are living in the right kind of ECM.

ECM is made of many molecules, including collagen proteins, which usually form long strands and add strength; laminin proteins, which help form sheets like basement membranes; and hyaluronic acid, a polysaccharide that holds water like a sponge, adds volume, and makes ECM gelatinous. Elastin is an ECM protein used for stretchiness, sort of the spandex of the cellular world. There are many others, but the upshot is that ECM contains hundreds of molecules, each with very different jobs.

ECM is made by cells. To do this, your cells secrete proteins and other molecules that assemble themselves into different shapes. Your cells can't construct ECM the way a person can build a piece of furniture. Instead, they spit out parts and rely on those parts to self-assemble spontaneously into the necessary structures. The self-assembly is passive, so the proteins and other components just bounce around until they hit something they have an affinity for. Like magnetic tiles that make it easy for kids to build castles, ECM molecules snap together under the right conditions.

Cells can also secrete enzymes that break down ECM, or specific ECM components. With cells producing and destroying ECM, you end up with a cycle known as ECM turnover. This allows cells to remodel and reshape tissues. For example, there are cells called osteoblasts and osteoclasts, which are continually creating and destroying your bones. This allows your bone ECM to be adapted to the demands you place on it. It's why an orthodontist can rearrange your teeth with braces. It's also why keeping up with exercise is so important to your health.

ECM varies widely between different tissues; just think of the compositional differences needed to produce the mechanical properties of the heart versus the stomach. That said, there are some common shapes and repeated patterns. A common pattern is a sheet that separates inside from outside. Your skin is an example, but the sheets are also used to create tubes like blood vessels. Lining the surface of the sheets are epithelial cells that help maintain the barrier. On the other side of the barrier are more cells and more ECM, but the arrangement is more complicated. Instead of a simple sheet with cells on top, you have a lattice of ECM proteins with different cells inside depending on the tissue.

The ECM does more than just provide places for cells to sit or move around. In addition to providing structure, ECM also has signaling properties that help direct cell behavior. The most direct is that cells can feel the mechanical properties of ECM. If they feel stiff, bone-like ECM, they will think they are on bone and act like it. This is good if they actually are on bone, but if your arteries are stiff it will cause problems. In addition to information transmitted to cells mechanically, signaling molecules are stored in ECM. When ECM is disrupted, cells will receive those signals and respond accordingly.

ECM Damage

ECM gets damaged over time, just like other structural materials can get damaged. If you have a thick metal wire, you can bend it relatively easily once. Bending it back is harder because the first bend damages the crystal structure of the wire, making it stiffer and weaker. If you bend it enough times, eventually the wire will snap in two. A similar process happens to components of your ECM.

When you're young, the ECM is soft where it needs to be soft, hard where it needs to be hard, resilient, and pure. Every year it gets slightly damaged, and strong, flexible collagen molecules in your skin become stiff and weak. Elastin proteins begin to fray like old bungee cords. Eventually, your bones can't handle the stress of a fall, and your arteries can't handle the pressure of your own heartbeat. The latter is particularly problematic, as small ruptures can cause little strokes that destroy brain tissue, and big ones can kill you.

ECM damage isn't all wear-and-tear. Cells can also damage ECM by laying down too much material or producing it in the wrong orientation. This happens when cells produce scars to try to heal wounds. Cells can also generate scar-like material throughout otherwise healthy tissue, making it stiff and fibrotic—a process termed fibrosis. This is a type of ECM damage that leads to a variety of diseases of old age: weakened lungs, stiffened arteries, dysfunctional kidneys, and damage to the brain.

So the components of ECM affect its function, and if these components are in the wrong quantities, the wrong positions, or themselves malformed, then the ECM won't work properly. Improperly constructed proteins, whether they have the wrong sequence of amino acids, are simply misfolded, or are in the wrong concentration, can cause problems for the ECM and the cells that depend on it. For example, if cells produce too many ECM-degrading enzymes, the excessive demolition will weaken the ECM. This is what happens with osteoporosis, which involves the deterioration of bone tissue.

ECM damage also interferes with brain maintenance processes. With age, the ECM around neurons becomes difficult to remodel, which can prevent neurons from adapting their behavior. This makes it harder for people to learn. Similarly, damaged ECM can make it difficult for the brain to produce new cells and for existing cells to keep the brain healthy. Similar processes might also impact the interaction of the central nervous system with the rest of the body, making it hard to keep organs like muscles functioning properly. If damaged ECM reduces the number of connections between your brain and your muscles, or weakens the signal for the connections you do have, then your muscles will be slower and weaker even if the muscle itself is the same.

One case where ECM damage is particularly harmful to cells is at stem cell niches. These are specialized locations where stem cells live. The ECM within the stem cell niche provides essential signals that help maintain stem cell identity and regulate their function. Without proper ECM cues, stem cells often lose their capacity for self-renewal. So, if they move away from the niche, or if the niche degrades or changes over time, it can lead to stem cell exhaustion and failure to supply the cells needed to maintain or repair tissue. For example, the stem cells that produce your blood cells have a cozy niche in the marrow inside your bones. If the bone marrow becomes inhospitable, it can lead to an insufficient supply or imbalance of different types of blood cells.

The upshot is that damage accumulation in your extracellular matrix limits your maximum lifespan. Once your ECM is damaged enough, nothing your cells do can keep you alive. This might also mean that ECM repair could be the key to breaking the current human lifespan records.

ECM is relatively understudied compared to cells and fluids. Perhaps for this reason, it has also been undervalued by the longevity community. While it's probably much more important to radical life extension than many people think, it's also probably much harder to rejuvenate than people believe. This combination means that it's worth spending time familiarizing yourself with how the ECM works, what technologies currently exist for testing and interacting with it, and what strategies could potentially return it to a youthful state. That's a lot to ask given the diversity of ECM components, the diversity of damage throughout all of them, and the relative lack of control cells have over ECM. It is probably worth the effort, though, because who knows what treasure is buried within the ECM.

Fluids

Along with cells and ECM, your body can't function without extracellular fluids. Fluids are used to move gases, nutrients, wastes, and heat around the body. They also protect joints, help organs maintain their shape, and lubricate surfaces for breathing, swallowing, and speech. Only about two-thirds of the water in your body is inside cells. The rest performs specialized functions in different tissues.

The most common extracellular fluid is interstitial fluid, which surrounds cells and permeates the extracellular matrix. Interstitial fluid is important for allowing nutrients and waste to be transferred between blood and cells. It also allows cells to properly secrete and take up signaling molecules.

The second most common is blood plasma. It's the liquid portion of blood that carries hormones, electrolytes, nutrients, and waste. It's critical for allowing the circulation of blood, maintaining blood pressure, and supporting immune responses.

There are also smaller amounts of specialized fluids like cerebrospinal fluid, synovial fluid, eye humors, and various lubricants. Cerebrospinal fluid cushions your brain and spinal cord, and helps remove waste from the central nervous system. Synovial fluid reduces friction and provides nutrients to cartilage in joints. The humors in the eyes help them maintain their shape and optical properties, as well as support nutrient and waste transport.

There are other fluids as well, but the important thing is not to memorize them all. Rather, try to get a sense of how fluids degrade with age.

Fluid Damage

Fluids are an important and underappreciated part of your body. Just like cells and ECM, fluids change dynamically to support tissue function. Also like cells and ECM, fluids change in detrimental ways as we get older.

One common type of damage to fluids is simply altered quantity. As we get older, we tend to have reduced blood plasma volume, which can lead to dangerous drops in blood pressure, for instance, after standing up. A lower volume of synovial fluid can reduce its protective effect on joints and contribute to osteoarthritis. Conversely, interstitial fluid can increase in volume as age-related changes impair drainage. This can contribute to problems like swollen ankles and congestive heart failure as fluid builds up in places it shouldn't be.

The viscosity of fluids can also change for the worse. For example, blood flow can become sluggish, which contributes to hypertension. Synovial fluid can become too thin or too viscous, reducing its ability to lubricate or nourish cartilage.

Changes in the composition of molecules being carried by the fluid can be problematic as well. Electrolyte imbalances in plasma or interstitial fluid can lead to cardiac arrhythmias, and this age-related imbalance usually won't be solved by chugging your favorite sports drink.

Oxidized molecules in fluids can also contribute to dysregulation of exposed cells. Pro-inflammatory factors also tend to rise with age, which is thought to contribute to many diseases, including diabetes.

Reduced turnover of fluids can lead to the accumulation of waste products. For example, reduced drainage of cerebrospinal fluid is thought to be a contributing factor to the accumulation of protein aggregates in the brain during neurodegenerative disease. This might be partially caused by the way the ECM around the brain changes with age, restricting the drainage of cerebrospinal fluid from the brain to the body. ECM damage can lead to fluid damage.

Age-related damage to fluids can also result from cellular dysfunction. One way cells can damage fluids is by excreting the wrong molecules. Cells spit out many different things, from atoms, to individual proteins, to little packages called extracellular vesicles. Your cells produce many kinds of extracellular vesicles, which can carry messages and spare parts to distant places within you. If cells send out the right proportion of the right molecules, your fluids will be healthier and they will keep your cells healthier. For example, your immune system fills your fluids with not just immune cells, but specialized molecules that kill pathogens. Antibodies are one type, but there are many others like the complement system, which consists of proteins that can work together to kill bacteria. All the various molecular tools and signals that cells secrete are called the secretome and, as we age, both the components and the composition of the secretome deteriorate.

For example, in an older individual, cells will secrete too many inflammatory signals. Your fluids will then carry them around and cause other cells to engage in actively harmful behaviors. Like a nursery full of crying babies, it's hard for immune cells to tell who is hungry, who is sick, and who is only crying because it's noisy. It makes it difficult for immune cells to go where they are most needed. Normally, infection or trauma causes acute inflammation to attract these cells, but in old age this signaling is masked by general inflammation.

This process is called inflammaging: the overactive inflammation associated with aging. Inflammaging leads immune cells to go from doing their jobs like professional security guards, without damaging healthy tissue much, to doing their jobs like amateur bounty hunters, and being less careful about what gets caught in the crossfire as they chase random signals from all over.

Common Patterns in Age-Related Damage

While damage varies widely across cells, ECM, and fluids, there are some common patterns that can be recognized.

At the molecular level, the simplest damage is loss of function in long-lived molecules. In cells, DNA is the longest lived molecule, and it loses function over time via mutations. In the ECM, a classic example is the protein elastin, which makes your skin and other tissues soft and bouncy. These molecules are primarily made in youth and slowly degrade over time, like old, dried-out rubber bands. As they wear down, your skin becomes wrinkly and fragile, your arteries become stiff, leading to high blood pressure, and your lungs have a harder time recoiling, which leads to shortness of breath, not to mention problems with your bladder and joints.

Another example is collagen molecules, which are structural proteins in most tissues. There's a wide variety of collagens, and whenever there aren't enough of them, tissue function can suffer. Structural support from collagen is essential for the shape and function of your organs, and loss of collagens can lead to poor wound healing, osteoporosis, joint instability, and injuries to tendons and ligaments. It also leads to cosmetic problems like fine lines in the skin, large pores, and general sagginess.

Long-lived molecular damage can occur in fluids as well, as seen in persistent organic pollutants like perfluorohexane sulfonate. These come from nonstick cookware and can stay in your blood for years.

Aside from general wear-and-tear, molecules often get damaged in similar ways whether they are inside a cell or outside of it. Common types of damage are oxidation, cross-linking, and, in the case of RNA and proteins, misfolding. Think of how easy it is to accidentally get a knot in a necklace or your hair and you'll appreciate how difficult it is to keep long RNAs and proteins coiled correctly.

RNAs and proteins can do cool things like binding to specific molecules, acting as enzymes, taking on structural roles, and so on, but only if they fold correctly. If they fold themselves into the wrong shape, they won't do their jobs and, at the very least, they will waste space and energy. Sometimes things are even worse, as a misfolded RNA or protein does something actively harmful whether they are inside cells, ECM, or fluids.

Two common problems due to misfolding are aggregation and prion-like behavior. When a protein folds, the hydrophobic parts tend to clump together in the center, and the hydrophilic parts stick out into the surrounding water. If a protein misfolds, then sometimes the hydrophobic parts are exposed and can stick to other proteins with the same problem. For example, you can have misfolded amyloid beta aggregates in the central nervous system, and these aggregates will encourage normal-shaped amyloid beta to misfold and subsequently aggregate as well.

For proteins that are less stable, having one misfolded protein can seed the random aggregation of other proteins of the same kind into clumps. One example is transthyretin, which commonly aggregates in the heart muscle and leads to weakening of the heart. You might think of this as Alzheimer's of the heart, but in fact this kind of aggregation happens in all of your tissues and organs as you age. For example, a protein called desmin can aggregate in skeletal muscles and cause similar problems. The same goes for keratin aggregation in the skin and liver.

Some proteins are even worse, as they directly cause other proteins to misfold. The classic example is the major prion protein; once this is misfolded, it takes on a shape that actively causes other prion proteins to take on the same dangerous shape. This spreads throughout an organism, usually destroying the nervous system and leading to death. It can infect other individuals or other species if the misfolded protein is transmitted, for instance through ingestion. This is what causes mad cow disease. Another example is alpha-synuclein, which spreads from cell to cell and causes Parkinson's disease.

Proteins don't need to misfold to misbehave. For example, there are protein complexes that regulate the traffic of molecules between the cell's nucleus and the cytoplasm. These are called nuclear pore proteins. They can become oxidized or cross-linked in ways that prevent them from maintaining the barrier, so stuff that's supposed to stay in the nucleus leaks out, and stuff that's supposed to stay outside leaks in. This is especially true for long-lived cells like neurons, because they can't use cell division as an opportunity to rebuild the nucleus with fresh parts.

You can also accumulate small molecules that interfere with biological function. One example is calcium deposits. This is often seen in the calcification of arteries and heart valves, which makes them stiff and increases the risk of cardiovascular disease.

When cells, ECM, and fluids combine into tissues and organs, we see new patterns of aging damage independent of the individual components. A common problem with advanced age is the redistribution of fat cells throughout the body. The fat cells may be healthy, but if you end up with fewer fat cells where they should be, and instead find them embedded in muscle tissue, surrounding organs, and so on, your body won't work as well. For example, as you get older, your thymus begins to lose the thymic cells that train your immune system; those cells are replaced with fat cells that effectively just sit on the couch and eat potato chips. This process is called thymic fatty involution, and it greatly decreases your immune system's ability to respond to both infections and vaccines. Fat is an essential part of the body, but in the wrong places it can make you sick.

At the organ level, aging leads to weakened muscles, a weaker immune system, weaker skin, weaker bones, and a slower, less effective brain, among other problems. Each of these, in turn, causes damage accumulation to accelerate throughout the body. Muscles normally provide structural support that protects our bodies, but they also have important metabolic and signaling functions. That's part of the reason why exercise is so good for you. You don't just improve your muscles, but every part of your body benefits from the chemical messages sent out by muscles when you use them. So muscle wasting leads to poor quality of life directly through reduced mobility, but also through impairment of other systems in the body.

Weakened skin ECM leads to increased infections and damaged cells. Damaged fat leads to metabolic disorders and inflammation in your bloodstream. Inflammatory factors in your blood lead to a weaker immune system and damaged ECM, and so on. There's no part of the body that uniquely drives aging, but damage does accumulate at different rates in different parts of the body for different people. Notably, ovaries go through a period of rapid aging before menopause. In general, every part of the body is damaged both by its own aging and by age-related changes in the rest of the body.

Key Takeaways

The human body is essentially a composition of cells, extracellular matrix, and fluids—each of which is itself a complex mix of proteins, sugars, fats, and nucleic acids. In each of them, hundreds of thousands of different types of proteins, noncoding RNAs, and other molecules are all bouncing around performing different tasks.

These are organized into tissues, organs, and systems that work together to keep you alive and healthy. The diverse cells, ECM molecules, and fluids have complex relationships that lead to an even greater variety of aging damage. Things can go wrong at many different levels, from the smallest molecule to the largest organs. In addition, age-related damage varies both by person and within individuals.

There's no single root cause when it comes to age-related disease because of the many feedback loops in human biology. Damage to your cells can cause them to damage your ECM. That ECM damage can then damage fluids. All of this happens in parallel as you age, so every part of you is contributing to dysfunction elsewhere while also getting interference from everywhere else.

All of this complex machinery works beautifully while you're young. Later things start to turn ugly. As we consider what to do about aging, we need to account for damage not only to cells, but also extracellular matrix and fluids. How can we slow the rate at which damage accumulates to each of them? How can we repair that damage and restore them all to a more youthful state?

There's no easy answer. The intricate details of human biology are currently beyond our understanding, and aging damage is even more opaque because it can alter each aspect of human biology in so many different ways. We don't have a complete map of cellular biochemistry, and even the rough sketches we do have are hard to comprehend. We have even less understanding of the extracellular matrix and extracellular fluids.

However, recognizing the size and complexity of the problem isn't a reason for despair. It's an indication of progress, because only when we admit how overwhelming the threat is do we have any chance of designing effective strategies against it. So rather than banking on an easy answer—or even a single hard one—let's admit that there are many obstacles and that our ignorance is vast, then make a plan that accounts for both. Don't bring a knife to a gunfight.

So given what we do know about aging, what would a good strategy look like?

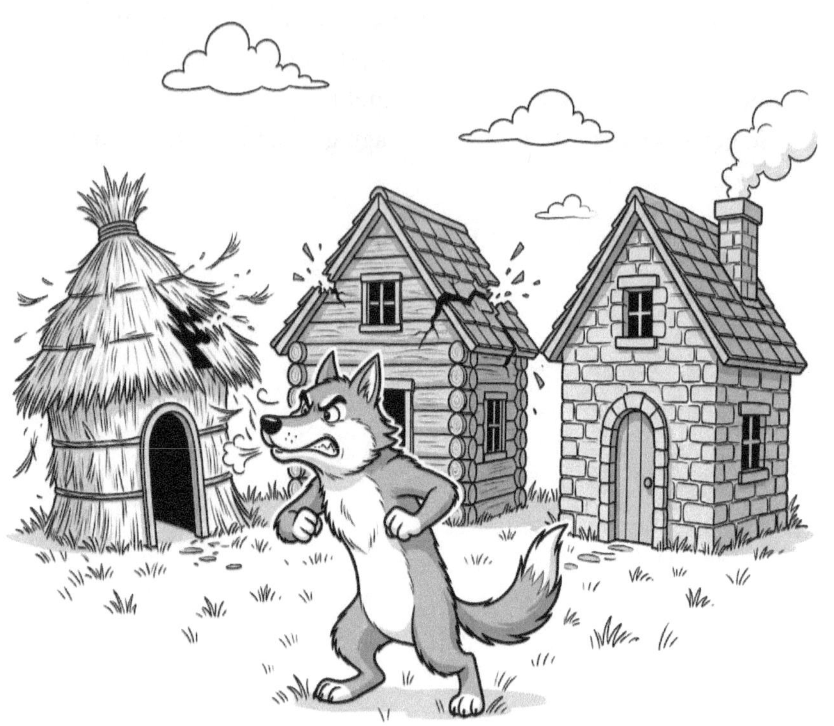

CHAPTER 5

BETTER STRATEGIES

We know we can't find a single cure for aging—there are just too many different problems. It would be equally misguided to try to find separate treatments for every age-related disease. Taking a reactive approach to the diseases of aging has led to beneficial medicines, but it has done little to meaningfully extend lifespan.

With such a big, convoluted problem, how can we hope to solve it? What we need are strategies that take what we currently know and put us in the best position to win. We need ways of making progress that neither require us to redesign human biology at the molecular level nor involve sweeping back the tide of geriatric diseases. We need to find alternative approaches that can have a big impact, and the sooner the better.

Better strategies don't need to be perfect plans. They don't need to have all the answers, or even a guarantee that they will work. They simply need to offer plausible shots at solving the problem in a reasonable time frame. A good strategy must be abstract enough to account for our ignorance, yet specific enough to direct resources toward the highest-value work. It should also give people immediately actionable steps. Most importantly, it must use every advantage we have to save time and, thereby, lives.

Simplifying the Problem

The first advantage we have is that we can simplify the problem. Age-related diseases are numerous, and most of them are dangerous, if not deadly. The diseases vary widely. They affect many different tissues and organs. We can sometimes treat the symptoms, and occasionally we can cure the disease completely, like when we resect a tumor. But there are too many diseases of aging to have any chance of curing them all, at least not anytime soon.

Fortunately, it appears that even though there are many age-related diseases, sets of them often have related underlying causes. For example, arterial plaques lead to both heart attacks and strokes. If a single type of damage can lead to multiple diseases, then treating that damage could be an efficient way to prevent or cure those diseases. In the previous case, we could address both problems by targeting plaques directly.

It very well could turn out to be faster and easier to target the upstream causes of age-related disease, rather than trying to develop individual therapies for age-related conditions after they occur. This is the main idea behind the geroscience hypothesis. Our bodies change in detrimental ways as we age, and this slow accumulation of age-related damage leads to dysfunction and disease. If we create technology to repair that damage, then the horde of diseases that afflict the elderly will be delayed and people will live longer, healthier lives.

Treating damage is both a preventative and curative approach because it targets upstream causes of diseases like cancer, cardiovascular disease, dementia, and metabolic disease. Approaches that go directly at diseases of aging may fix the proximate cause of a patient's suffering, like the example of cutting out a tumor. However, the common cause and greatest risk factor for age-related diseases is aging itself. That means the intensity and frequency of these diseases will only get worse over time. By moving our efforts earlier in the process, we can not only do a better job treating conditions, but we can also potentially prevent them in the first place.

It's much better to remove plaques from your arteries than to try to fix the aftermath of a stroke. It's better to destroy cells that have cancerous mutations before they can evolve and spread throughout the body. Unfortunately, many companies are still working on treating age-related diseases rather than aging. They will hopefully help some people live a little longer, but they are unlikely to help the vast majority of people greatly extend their lives.

Part of the reason is that, with our current level of understanding, we can only make small adjustments to biological processes, and even then they often lead to unintended consequences. Many people have died because a drug that was supposed to help in one area of our biology ended up being toxic in another. So it should be no surprise that we're nowhere near being able to solve aging by re-engineering our biology. Fortunately, we don't have to.

The geroscience hypothesis suggests that many diseases can be treated or even prevented by targeting a more manageable array of age-related damage. This requires us to address upstream causes of disease, but it doesn't require us to go all the way upstream and contend with the root causes of aging. Damage is an intermediary between metabolism and disease and, by targeting age-related damage, you can both treat diseases more effectively and avoid the complexity of trying to tinker with metabolism.

So the second advantage is that, just as we can simplify the problem by focusing on damage instead of diseases, we can also simplify the solution by focusing on damage instead of metabolism. For example, cancer has many different causes including DNA repair defects that raise mutation rates, deactivated tumor suppressor genes, and escape from replication limits, among others. You could try to change human biology so these things don't happen, and that would certainly cure cancer. However, the effort required seems unrealistic in the foreseeable future. What seems more realistic is finding ways to repair the damage after it happens, for example by detecting cells that have dangerous mutations and clearing them from the body.

It will usually be easier to fix damage than to prevent it from occurring, just as it's much easier to occasionally wipe your shoes than to keep them from getting dirty in the first place. We'll make faster progress if we accept that damage is inevitable and focus on removing the damage, either by repairing it or replacing damaged cells and tissues. This matters because you could spend all the money in the world trying to understand and modify human biology without creating a single therapy.

The same is true downstream: fighting diseases of aging one at a time would only have a marginal impact on lifespan. Curing all cancers would add only a few years to average lifespan, because as people get older, we're continually finding new ways that human biology can go awry. Each type of aging damage is like a time bomb. Allow it to stick around long enough and some deadly manifestation will present itself. DNA mutations will kill you eventually, either through cancer or through inactivation of essential genes. Intracellular aggregates will kill you eventually, because cells that don't divide will stop working when they fill up with junk. Extracellular aggregates will kill you eventually, because tissue that's stiff and brittle will break and destroy the organ systems that you depend on for survival.

Each of these enemies can kill you in different ways. There are hundreds of types of cancer. There are many ways that protein aggregates can stop your heart, lungs, or brain from working properly. So while beating aging damage is a multi-faceted problem, beating aging diseases one at a time is orders of magnitude more difficult. Of course, it's valuable to find treatments for age-related disease, especially for those who already have the disease, but every day spent on them is a missed opportunity to develop treatments for upstream causes. The closer you can get to root causes, the more people you can help, and the more durable the benefits will be.

The upshot is that complex biology leads to relatively simple damage, which then leads to complex diseases. By targeting aging damage, we should find ways to treat many diseases. Also by targeting damage, we can avoid wild goose chases through human biology. So targeting damage leads to huge gains in both efficiency and effectiveness by avoiding both upstream and downstream complexities.

Downstream in the realm of age-related disease lies an endless amount of work that will have little impact on radical life extension in general, but may be important to you or to people you care about. Upstream are opportunities that could be hugely beneficial for radical life extension and could have a massive impact on large numbers of people, but they will usually be very difficult to capitalize on.

It might be tempting to try to stop the aging process in the first place, but that would require technology that's far beyond anything we have today. It would require engineering control over all of the biological pathways of the body, many of which are currently unmapped. Control means not just being able to understand and modify, but also to create new biology that's superior to what we currently have—a daunting task.

Instead, the damage-repair approach to radical life extension was developed by Aubrey de Grey and popularized through his 2007 book, Ending Aging. It identifies common types of aging damage and ideas for repairing them—focusing on technological development in specific areas that are understood well enough for us to make progress. Yet, developing damage repair therapies comprehensive enough to radically extend lifespan is still a massive undertaking, and may take more time than most or all of us have left. Are there any other ways to make things easier?

Longevity Escape Velocity

There's one more way to simplify the problem: by leveraging the nonlinear effects of incremental progress. If we had to completely solve aging before we got any benefits, that would be bad news. If longevity technology only produced one-time benefits, that would also spell trouble. However, creating therapies that can repair aging damage leads to benefits that accumulate over time.

This is because removing damage does more than cure disease. It resets the state of the damaged system back to more youthful levels.

Your systems are highly interconnected, and rejuvenation of any one of them benefits all of them, making them more robust and effective. Remember, curing one age-related disease while leaving the damage merely sets you up to die a little later from the next age-related disease. By contrast, therapies that remove damage delay age-related disease in general, buying you more time than curing a specific disease alone. Damage repair also makes it easier to treat age-related diseases when they do happen, improving your odds of survival and benefiting from the next wave of technologies.

While current medicine can extend your lifespan, damage-repair therapies could achieve even greater gains. In a world where many people live longer on average, many more would make it to their 100th birthday. Those who become centenarians one year will tend to be healthier and live longer lives than those who turned 100 the previous year, simply because of technological progress. This virtuous cycle will lead to a situation where people who live long enough enter a phase in which longevity technology begins to greatly extend lifespans.

Today, by some estimates, technological progress adds a month or two to your life every year. So each decade you survive, you would expect to gain an extra year or more. However, technological progress is accelerating, so the amount of time you gain each year might increase over time. At some point, each year you live will let you live an additional six months. So, just by surviving a decade, you will get to add five years to your life.

Eventually this reaches a tipping point. Once technology is advanced enough, life expectancy will rise by one year each year. That means drugs, therapies, devices, and other medical technology will be keeping you at a level of health where your risk of death doesn't increase over time. This is called longevity escape velocity (LEV); once you reach it, you're unlikely to die of old age. Technology could thus theoretically continue to outpace biological aging and age-related decline. Historically, we've raised average lifespan faster than maximum—a measure of how hard this is, not proof it can't be done, and partly the result of never having targeted aging directly. The principle stands: technology can outpace aging.

Surviving to the point of LEV would radically extend your lifespan. But what if that inflection point is expected to happen after your life expectancy? Does that mean there's no hope for you? Actually, there's still reason for hope. That's because the closer you get to that critical point, the more your life will be extended by medical technology.

Suppose that in the decade before LEV is achieved, technology goes from extending lifespans by six months to extending them by 12 months. That means over those 10 years you gained an additional seven and a half years of life. So technology that was 10 chronological years away was only two and a half biological years away. This effect helps more and more the better technology gets, increasing your chance of being caught in the wave of longevity technology and being propelled to LEV. So the age you need to survive to might be much more attainable than you expect. Exponential curves are counterintuitive, but consider the change that has occurred over your lifetime in computational technology. What if a similar acceleration occurred in medical technology?

This kind of nonlinear effect is hard to imagine, so consider an analogy. Suppose you're on a boat with 10 days' worth of food. To survive, you need to sail to an island, but the island is far away. Normally it would take you 20 days to get to the island. However, this island has a strange weather pattern such that the closer you get, the stronger the winds are pushing you toward the island. If the winds stayed constant, you would not make it, but since the winds push you faster and faster the closer you approach, it gets easier and easier to get there. On the first day you travel only 5% of the distance to the island, but on the tenth day you travel the final 20%. You make it before you run out of food because of this acceleration. Similarly, technological acceleration could help a surprising number of people reach LEV.

So there's some reason for hope, despite not knowing when LEV will occur. However, this technological turning point is more of a process than a single breakthrough event. No one has yet pushed human lifespan much past its current ceiling, and damage repair is probably what it will take—though we won't know for certain until we try, and we've only just barely started.

Slowing Damage Versus Repairing Damage

Once you center your thinking on damage, you can consider how to deal with it. One approach is to reduce the rate at which damage is produced. The other is to repair the damage after it has occurred.

For example, there are already drugs that can slow the progression of age-related damage. Statins can retard the accumulation of plaque in your arteries, so instead of plaques growing 2% each year, maybe they only grow 1%. On the other hand, a drug that reversed plaque size by 1% could be taken each year to get a similar effect. In either case, you live longer and delay age-related disease.

Other things being equal, damage repair is superior in that it brings you back to a younger state. This makes you healthier, and the extra time you buy is healthier too. By contrast, reducing the rate of damage accumulation will, at best, keep you as healthy as you currently are. Staying the same is great if you are still young, but billions of people are already suffering from aging. Prevention would come too late for them, but repair would work for everyone.

Reversing damage also has the advantage that it can be done periodically. It doesn't matter if your plaque growth rate is 2% if every year you can reset it to zero. Therapies can be timed to match the rate of damage accumulation, so fast damage might be reversed every year, while slower damage only requires treatment every 10 years. This kind of repair has the potential to stave off aging indefinitely if the effect sizes are large and comprehensive enough.

In many cases, it may be easier to reverse damage than to prevent it. For example, it's hard to prevent cells from becoming senescent because they are supposed to do just that in certain situations to protect the body. Yet, it's relatively straightforward to clear senescent cells with drugs, and such therapies are already in various stages of development. So why do a lot of work to prevent cellular senescence when it's easier and more convenient to repair the problem after the fact?

In other situations, it might seem easier to slow the aging process than it is to reverse the damage once it has been done. There will probably be instances where damage is hard to repair, but slowing damage accumulation is relatively easy. For example, it might be extremely difficult to repair arbitrary DNA mutations with gene therapies, but it may be relatively tractable to lower the mutation rate by improving DNA maintenance. So while prevention is less valuable than repair in general, it might make sense in some cases to pursue low-hanging fruit in the realm of preventing damage from occurring.

For any particular kind of damage, therapies for reversal may come before or after methods for prevention. This is partly because slowing damage and repairing damage require different technical approaches. If you want to reduce the rate of damage accumulation, you need to understand how it's produced and modify that process. You can search through human metabolism and look for pathways that produce damage, and then design ways to alter them favorably. If you want to reduce the amount of damage, you only need to understand what the damage is and repair it. As a result, slowing damage will often require more upfront work for the same level of benefit.

The contrast between slowing and repairing damage also comes down to how much time each buys you. If your goal is radical life extension, you should not care too much about how we get there. If one strategy gets you more time, then that strategy has an advantage.

For some people who otherwise would not have made the cut, therapies that merely slow aging may allow them to reach longevity escape velocity. When a cure for cancer is developed, it will help people live a few more years on average. That may seem small but, to marginal people, those years are precious. It may allow them to live until the next breakthrough. For example, if they live long enough to see a cure for cardiovascular disease, that could get them a few more years. And so on with the major causes of death. Each time you do that, you reach future technology that can take care of aging more effectively. The future is the safest place to be.

Slowing aging and reversing aging are both valid and can be pursued in parallel. Just be clear about which strategy you're considering at any particular moment so that you can accurately weigh the costs and benefits. An opportunistic approach may lead to faster gains and better outcomes for those who are alive today, while pursuing the most difficult therapies in each category might unnecessarily keep you and others in mortal danger.

Improving Average Versus Maximum Lifespan

The problem of maximum lifespan is related to preventing damage and repairing damage. Your risk of dying goes up exponentially with age, meaning the more damage you have, the more likely you are to get a critical failure in one of your systems and die. This currently creates a kill zone around the age of 115 that people don't live through. You may wonder if there's some fundamental reason that humans can't live beyond that. If that were the case, perhaps the best that advanced technology could do would be to make people relatively healthy until they are around that age, and then people would die from a catastrophic failure, with countless things going awry around the same time.

This is effectively the case with current approaches to treating age-related diseases. Modern medicine does little to change maximum lifespan, but it does a good job keeping you alive longer than you otherwise would have been. More people are living longer on average but the maximum, as far as we can tell, isn't changing. Certainly a 10-year shift in average lifespan has not led to a proportional shift at centenarian ages. Taken to the extreme, conventional modern medicine might eventually help everyone live to around 110 years old, but in such poor health that they would die shortly after. Charts that show survival by age look like a smooth downward curve, but this would be "squaring the curve" into a cliff-edge.

Longevity technology does something different. Instead of treating symptoms to keep you going a little longer, it treats the underlying mechanisms to make you younger. If you develop technology that slows aging, then you stretch out the curve and increase maximum lifespan. If you develop technology that reverses aging, you effectively move back along the curve, pushing the maximum out even further.

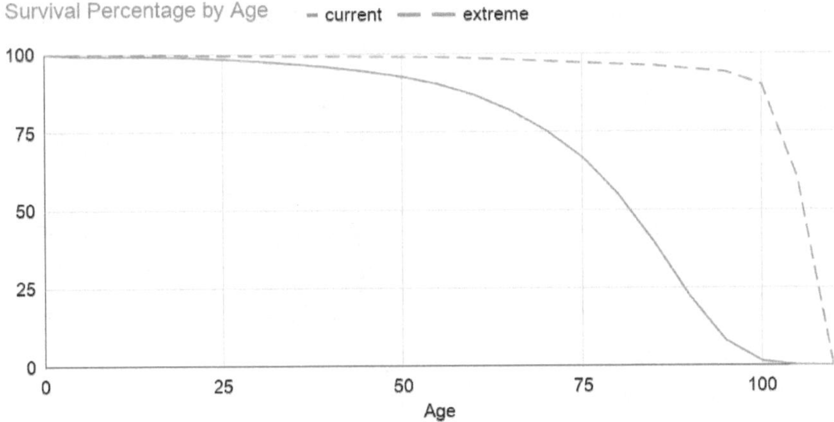

Extending healthspan without extending lifespan shifts mortality to later years.

So, on one hand, you can develop technology that makes people live longer without giving them extra healthy years of life. This is what happens when someone who is cured of cancer gets an extra five years that they otherwise would not have had, but those years are fraught with illness and poor quality of life. On the other hand, you can develop technology that makes people live both longer and in better health. For instance, a drug that reduced the rate of age-related muscle loss would give people both longer and healthier lives.

This has been observed in studies of centenarians. Those who live to extreme old age aren't typically the people who survive terrible illnesses, but those who avoid them altogether by chance or lucky genetics.

An extended healthspan is nice because it means a higher quality of life. Nobody likes the idea of becoming more and more decrepit, losing independence, and eventually being unable to enjoy many of the things that make life great. That's not to mention that the more damaged your body becomes and the more chronic diseases you have, the more likely you are to die. So healthspan extension is an important part of what the longevity community is trying to do. However, some approaches to extending healthspan may not impact lifespan much, in which case the goal of radical life extension isn't achieved.

There's nothing in biology that sets a universal limit on maximum lifespan. Other animals, like the Greenland shark, can live for several hundred years, and there seems to be no reason why humans could not enjoy radically longer lifespans with sufficiently advanced technology.

The steep drop-off at the end of life is an artifact of both human biology and the current state of technology. As various types of damage are retarded or repaired, new limits will be set for maximum lifespan. But eventually, each barrier will fall and people will live not only longer, but more healthily into the new old age.

We don't know when longevity technology will mature, so you want to make good decisions around risk and benefit. If an overly long-term view means that the indefinite solution to aging occurs after you die, you won't be around to enjoy it. More commonly, though, people take an overly short-term view, and put their efforts into buying small amounts of extra time with lifestyle interventions. Putting effort into your lifestyle is a good idea, so long as you're also supporting the development of therapies that target aging damage. Otherwise, you're just delaying the inevitable.

Another reason to focus on damage repair is that the first complete solution will probably only arise out of a variety of strategies and technologies in combination. If some silver bullet never comes, continual, hard-won gains may be the only path forward. This piecemeal approach only works if you're engaging with damage on some level. There are too many age-related diseases to stop them all. But by repairing damage, you can alleviate entire categories of age-related disease, and help your body function at a healthier, more youthful level. We want things that turn back the clock.

Of course, as long as any type of damage continues to accumulate, there will be some limit to maximum lifespan. The technology that helps people live to 130 years may not be enough to help people live to 150. But each obstacle only comes after a certain amount of time—time that can be used to invent new solutions.

Some people are currently reaching the first ceiling, but most people don't even get close to that. So, except for the exceptionally lucky, therapies that increase average lifespan are needed. Fortunately, by focusing on damage, we will probably improve both average and maximum lifespan at the same time.

In any case, if your goal is to live long enough to benefit from radical life extension technology, you'll need to consider factors that affect both lifespan and healthspan. The longer you remain healthy and disease free, the longer your lifespan is likely to be. But without some fundamental shift in technology, the end will be the same.

This brings us to one final way to simplify the problem, which is to decide who you are trying to develop a strategy for. Strategies will vary by personal circumstance and solving aging for one person is difficult enough, let alone trying to save everyone. For example, a pill designed for preventing damage will be more helpful for a young person than an old person. An older person has a higher level of accumulated damage, so their risk of dying will remain high even without additional damage accumulation.

Therapy type isn't the only consideration; timing matters too. Depending on your point of view, it may be more urgent to work on therapies that treat age-related diseases in people in their 70s and 80s, or to tackle the problems that prevent almost everyone from living beyond 115 years.

Potential Solutions

We have narrowed the scope of the problem by shifting attention away from biological drivers of aging that are hard to change, as well as chronic diseases of aging that are hard to treat, to aging damage. By focusing instead on ways to slow and reverse it, we can now start to think about solutions.

There are four potential strategies for radical life extension, each of which involves a different technological approach to the problem. The first is traditional pharmaceuticals, where you develop drugs that influence human biology through direct molecular interactions. The second is advanced bioengineering, where you develop gene therapies that can radically alter human biology with new genetic instructions. The third is replacement, where you substitute healthy body components for aged ones. The fourth is biostasis, where you put human biology on pause until future medical technology can reverse aging.

Each approach has its own set of advantages and disadvantages, which should be considered when deciding how best to use them.

Traditional Drug Development as a Strategy

The traditional pharma approach would be to use small molecules to treat aging. Small molecules are just what they sound like, molecules that are small enough to diffuse throughout the body and into cells. Common examples include aspirin and amoxicillin. So you would pick some area of biology that seems relevant to aging and then try to develop a small molecule drug that can have some positive effect on it. You would do this many times for different aspects of aging, and then combine them in a smart way into a cocktail that keeps you young and healthy as long as you take it.

Small molecule drugs are an old paradigm that has some advantages and several serious drawbacks. One big advantage is that it's easy to get them to where they need to go. Typically, you can take them orally and they will spread throughout the body.

They are also relatively easy to manufacture and distribute around the world. There's a large ecosystem of research labs and manufacturers that can produce small molecule drugs. There are established testing methodologies and regulatory pathways. Most of the drug development in the world goes toward small molecules. All of this makes it tempting to try to use small molecules for every problem. However, small molecule drugs have many disadvantages as well.

One is that they are difficult to develop. They require an understanding of molecular biology and metabolic pathways. This means spending a lot of time and money on research for each potential drug. It also means lots of testing, including long clinical trials, to determine whether a drug is safe and effective. The requirement to understand human biology deeply is part of what makes small molecules slow and costly to develop.

Despite all the work that goes into making them, they are relatively simple tools. They can influence existing cellular behaviors, or they can help interfere with, enhance, or destroy molecules in the body. They also degrade or are excreted over time, so they require regular redosing. This dosing has to be highly tuned to maintain the efficacy of the drug while avoiding toxicity.

However, the most problematic drawback of small molecules is that they have side effects. A drug might help with one problem, but cause other problems. This can be a good trade-off for acute diseases, but not for aging, where you have many different problems to solve.

As small molecules are specific to an individual problem, you would need many drugs to treat aging. Taking so many drugs will not only interfere with your normal bodily processes, but will also cause the drugs to interfere with each other, making them less effective and potentially leading to toxicity. So, in the fight against aging, small molecules need to be used sparingly. This limitation can already be seen in the elderly, who tend to have several chronic diseases and have to be careful about how the different medications they are prescribed interact.

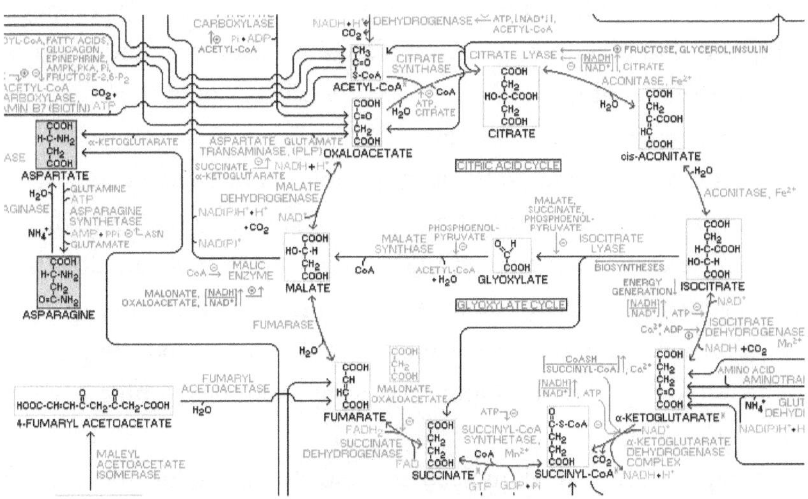

A diagram showing a small part of human metabolism.

The difficulty of trying to manipulate human biology is an important concept to internalize. Human metabolism is incredibly complex and intertwined. Here is a picture of a very small part of it.

Much of drug development focuses on understanding biological pathways like the ones above and modulating them with drugs. However, changing any small part of this can have unpredictable and dire consequences for an individual. Drugs have side effects, and the hundreds of drugs it would take to try to stop aging would lead to many unpleasant side effects. That's not to mention the uncomfortable feeling of eating hundreds of pills each morning.

Of course, this approach has led to beneficial drugs for specific diseases and specific circumstances. Epinephrine auto-injectors can save the life of someone having an allergic reaction, and steroids can help in a variety of emergency and nonemergency situations. Antibiotics have been enormously beneficial for helping people live longer. But the time it would take to fully understand metabolic networks and then bring them under control with drugs is far beyond the lifetime of anyone alive today. It may not even be possible, given the difficulty of producing small molecules that can do only what you need them to do and nothing else.

In general, we know that simple drugs will be unable to achieve things like DNA mutation repair, or repair every type of ECM damage, among other necessary tasks. Even if small molecules could address every type of damage, the cumulative side effects would likely exceed what a person could safely tolerate.

Small molecules should be used sparingly, and mostly when their properties or the damage target give some compelling reason to do so. They can be developed against high value targets that can slow the accumulation of age-related damage or potentially reverse a few specific types of damage. At best, they are another tool in the toolbox. In general, though, they take time and attention away from developing higher-impact technology.

Examples of how small molecules could slow aging include helping to improve the transcription and translation processes, which falter with age. They might reverse aging by, for example, helping to clear extracellular and intracellular aggregates. They might help clear cells that have become senescent. But, even if you can do something with a small molecule, you should stop and consider if there might not be a better solution using more advanced bioengineering techniques.

Advanced Bioengineering as a Strategy

By contrast, advanced bioengineering could be a much more powerful tool in the quest for radical life extension. With bioengineering techniques, we can alter our genes, borrow beneficial genes from other species, or even design entirely new genetic programs for our cells to run. The effects of gene therapy can be controlled much more precisely than those of small molecule drugs. They can be used transiently, as in the case of mRNA therapies, integrated into the genome for lifelong expression, or designed to activate and deactivate with internal and external signals just like your own metabolic pathways.

Bioengineering can be used to generate a huge range of useful molecules within the body. Cells can be instructed to produce RNAs and proteins such as antibodies and enzymes to do useful work. Your body can become a precision medicine factory with the right genetic instructions. Many side effects of drugs would be eliminated if your cells produced them only exactly when and where they are needed, and nowhere else.

Even more powerfully, cells can be upgraded with improved characteristics, like resistance to viruses or anti-cancer mechanisms. They can be given instructions to make them more effective in their jobs, or to avoid bad behaviors that cause age-related damage. Cells can even be instructed to heal themselves somewhat, by giving them new aging damage repair machinery that can clear the damage that has accumulated—which would effectively make them younger.

Given enough time and effort, advanced bioengineering can become a complete solution for aging. However, as a strategy it has its own drawbacks. The biggest is that, like traditional pharmaceutical development, it requires a deep understanding of human biology to implement. It isn't a simple thing to make changes to cellular metabolic pathways. One gene can affect many parts of the cell and many processes within it. Not only that, but altering one cell's behavior can impact the behavior of neighboring cells and even distant cells in the body through signaling molecules. The second biggest problem is that we don't have the technology to safely and effectively change the human genome. Today, gene therapies are limited to simple diseases where modifying only a tiny percentage of your cells is sufficient to benefit the recipient— a far cry from what would be needed to tackle aging.

These two problems mean that advanced bioengineering will be a relatively slow and expensive road to radical life extension.

Replacement as a Strategy

Another approach that could be a complete solution to the problem of aging is replacement. Replacement means swapping in healthy body components for those that are damaged or lost. These could be molecules, cells, or even tissues and organs. One advantage of replacement is that it completely solves problems with whatever components are replaced. If your heart is fibrotic, necrotic, cancerous, or all three, then putting in a new one will solve these problems and more. The second advantage of replacement is that it doesn't require a detailed understanding of human biology to use. You simply find a spare part, swap it in, and thereby remove age-related damage and other diseases.

Replacement happens every day in normal clinical practice. People get bone marrow transplants, organ transplants, prosthetics, and more. There's a long history of using replacement to treat disease, and it holds great promise for treating aging.

However, replacement has several disadvantages. The first is that it can be difficult to find replacement parts. There's a long waiting list for organs to transplant, and many people die before they can get one. A second disadvantage is that, even if you have access to spare parts, it might be difficult or dangerous to swap them for the aged ones in your body. Even with modern technology, many people die from transplant surgeries.

So, while replacement isn't a perfect solution, it has the advantage that it doesn't have large scientific barriers and can theoretically restore any part of the body to youth and good health.

Biostasis as a Strategy

The final strategy for dealing with aging is biostasis. Biostasis isn't just a strategy for preventing damage, but perhaps the ultimate strategy. The idea is to take people who are dying and can't be saved by modern medicine, and give them a chance to benefit from future medical technology. It does this by either using cold temperatures or chemicals to freeze the molecules of their bodies in place. This prevents them from changing over time, including accumulating additional damage. With luck, the cardiovascular diseases and cancers that killed them will have a cure in the not-too-distant future.

Unlike the damage you accumulate while you're alive, the rate of damage to your body after your heart stops beating goes up dramatically. People can be brought back with CPR in the first few minutes, but the longer you go without circulation, the more difficult it is to revive you. So biostasis is best done immediately upon declaration of legal death to preserve your body in the best possible state, making it easier for the CPR of the future to bring you back. How long it will take to develop that technology is uncertain but, if you're in biostasis, you could theoretically wait for centuries without changing.

Biostasis, like replacement, doesn't require a deep understanding of human metabolism to implement—it's more of an engineering problem. Its biggest advantage, though, is that we already have the technology to perform the preservation process on people who need it.

The biggest drawback is that there's currently no technology that can revive someone from biostasis, and it isn't clear when, if ever, that technology will become available. The second is that you have no agency, so you'll be completely reliant on good caretaking from whatever organization is keeping you in stasis. The final drawback is that even if you manage to reverse the process, you still need to cure whatever killed you in the first place, be it aging or something else.

Still, biostasis is a reasonable approach to the problem and an essential tool in your toolkit for radical life extension.

Comparing Strategies

The four strategies discussed above can be divided in two ways. The first is whether they can cure aging, or whether they merely buy time. Bioengineering and replacement are complete solutions, while pharma and biostasis buy time. The second is whether they require the time and effort to deeply investigate human biology, or whether they are more of an engineering problem and thus relatively fast and easy to implement. On this metric, pharma and bioengineering require deep scientific knowledge while replacement and biostasis are more straightforward.

The first key takeaway from this is that time and resources intended for longevity should shy away from pharma and favor more complete solutions like bioengineering and replacement, as well as more cost-

	Understand Aging	**Bypass Aging**
Solve Aging	**Advanced Bioengineering**	**Replacement**
Buy Time	**Traditional Pharma**	**Biostasis**

Comparing the benefits and scientific cost of four strategies.

effective solutions like replacement and biostasis. The second key takeaway is that replacement is uniquely positioned as the strategy that could be a complete solution, but also gets a shortcut around the biggest obstacles of human biology.

The differences are striking. The amount of time that pharmaceutical products could buy you is on the order of 10 years, while the amount of time biostasis could buy you is hundreds of years. Not only is the benefit lopsided, but the work involved is as well. The time and money required to implement pharma solutions could be hundreds of billions over decades, while biostasis might be perfected in half the time for a fraction of the cost.

Similarly, the differences between the complete solutions are vast. The costs of implementing a solution to aging with bioengineering could be in the trillions of dollars over multiple decades, while the cost of a replacement solution would be closer to tens of billions over a single decade.

Strategies also differ in how broad an impact they can have. Small molecule and gene therapies each do one thing, so you need many of them. Biostasis and replacement can affect large volumes of tissue and all associated problems at once. Other things being equal, maybe it would be better to work on approaches that can have broad impact. Remember that aging is a combination of highly varied problems, so being able to cast a wide net will be highly beneficial.

So, is pharma really not a good place to spend your time and capital? Well, if your goal is to die wealthy, then pharma could be a perfectly good way to go. But if your goal is radical life extension, then your bias should be to avoid small molecule development unless some unusual opportunity presents itself. This is even more true for supplements, which have even less chance of helping with longevity, but can be brought to the market quickly. It doesn't matter how fast you can get a product to people if it doesn't do anything.

To be fair, small molecules have more potential than supplements. If you're particularly good at small molecule development or have experience with traditional biopharma finance, then perhaps you can make a difference in that field. Just make sure you're working on products that at least have the potential to meaningfully extend human lifespan. There are many, many drugs that you could spend 10 years bringing to market that might never make it through clinical trials, or have zero life extension potential even if they did.

If you absolutely must work in pharma, there are better and worse strategies within that space. First, you should try to use small molecules to target aging damage directly, rather than trying to improve healthspan and lifespan indirectly. Second, you should pick targets where small molecules have an advantage over bioengineering. While genetic medicines can produce proteins or cells that do almost anything, it can be hard to get them to every part of the body. Small molecules are currently better for getting to hard-to-reach places.

One category of aging damage for which small molecules could help is chemical cross-linking. Cross-links are chemical bonds that form between different molecules, sticking them together and deactivating or altering the function of the affected molecules. A common example is glucosepane, which is the result of sugar molecules cross-linking with the collagen in your skin, arteries, and more. The cross-links cause your tissues to become stiff and eventually lead to other problems.

Enzymes have been developed that can break glucosepane. Unfortunately, the cross-links are buried inside insoluble collagen fibers, so it's difficult for the enzymes to reach them. If a small molecule could be developed that selectively broke glucosepane, or merely provided a safe way to prevent it from forming, this might be one of the greatest contributions to longevity that a small molecule could make.

Beyond pharma, how should one think about the relative importance of the major strategies of biostasis, replacement, and bioengineering? Given the enormous amount of money already going into bioengineering, you should be biased toward investing time and money into biostasis and replacement. Given that biostasis is the only option that currently exists, if someone you care about has a short time horizon, then biostasis might win out over a full solution like replacement.

Conversely, if you believe that a bioengineering solution to aging could happen soon, then it might make sense to put all your eggs in that basket. A genetic medicine that produced life extension could be quickly ramped up and delivered to every person in the world, whereas biostasis and replacement would scale more slowly.

There are other factors to consider. For instance, biostasis can't rejuvenate you at all, while replacement can get you back to where you were. However, bioengineering can actually improve you. Enhancements aren't just a nice-to-have, but could meaningfully improve your chances of radical life extension. For example, with replacement you might get a new heart. But with bioengineering, you could have a heart that's resistant to heart attacks, infection, and other problems. It would actually last longer than your natural heart and help keep the rest of your body healthy as well.

But if your goal is to produce a solution to aging as quickly as possible, then replacement is where it is at. Maybe this should not be surprising, because replacement is the closest strategy to what billions of years of evolution came up with. Aging is a collection of complex problems and, over long enough time scales, basically everything that can go wrong will go wrong. Evolution has solved this problem by discarding old bodies and creating fresh, healthy ones through reproduction. Old adults produce young babies, so nature has mechanisms for rejuvenation that we can learn from.

First, individual cells have more options than multicellular organisms. A cell can focus on itself rather than playing a specialized role to support an organism. This allows it to recycle a large portion of its proteins and other molecules for new ones. It can also reset its epigenetic program, sort of like restarting a computer.

Second, a single cell can be free of any accumulated extracellular matrix damage. All of the new collagen, elastin, and other ECM components that it produces will be young and healthy. Adults can't do this because our survival depends on the continuing function of tissues, which require supporting ECM. If we could grow new ECM and move our cells onto it, we would live a lot longer. But that isn't practically feasible with current technology.

Third, a cell can dilute any internal damage through cell division. If a zygote has a bit of molecular garbage built up inside, then after it splits into two cells it only has half as much, then a quarter, and so on. But the cells of the zygote will divide 42 times before a baby is born, so the cells of the newborn will only have about a trillionth of any damage that was in the original cell. The solution to pollution is dilution.

The trick here is that it doesn't matter what kind of damage has accumulated. All damage is reduced and, even if you have a million different kinds, you still end up with young, healthy tissue. And you never have to understand what went wrong. There's something elegant about a solution that can reverse almost any kind of aging damage you throw at it.

Adults can't do any of these things, and it would be very difficult to make medications that have the same effects. So what hope is there of accomplishing a similar task for those who are alive today? It turns out that there are techniques under development to completely refresh cells, ECM, and fluids. Using these approaches, we can break the cycle and help restore vigor to adults that was previously only accessible to the young. Pushing this strategy to the limit could solve aging entirely.

Key Takeaways

There are three primary strategies for radical life extension: biostasis, replacement, and advanced bioengineering. These are not only plausible paths to radical life extension, but they are also the only hope for people living today. Nothing else will work.

Biostasis is the first strategy that can have a meaningful impact, probably followed by replacement in the near term, with bioengineering having the longest time horizons. Unfortunately, this is the opposite order to how desirable the therapies are. We would all prefer to get some gene therapy that keeps us 25 years old forever. And being frozen for 100 years beats being dead, but otherwise isn't that appealing. Regardless, we need to be realistic about these timelines if we want to rationally allocate our time and resources.

Of course, we can work on all three areas in parallel and see how quickly we can make progress. Different people will find their interests and skills more aligned with one than the others. Moreover, different people will need different combinations of each strategy to survive. So, we should continually update our estimates of how important each area is, and how important our contributions to each area could be.

To do that, you will need to have a deep understanding of the theory and practice of each strategy. Only once you're intimately familiar with how cryonics companies protect people, how organ transplantation cures disease, and how bioengineering can change the rules of the game of life, will you be ready to decide what works for you. And no matter what you choose, you'll be working on something that has a chance of working.

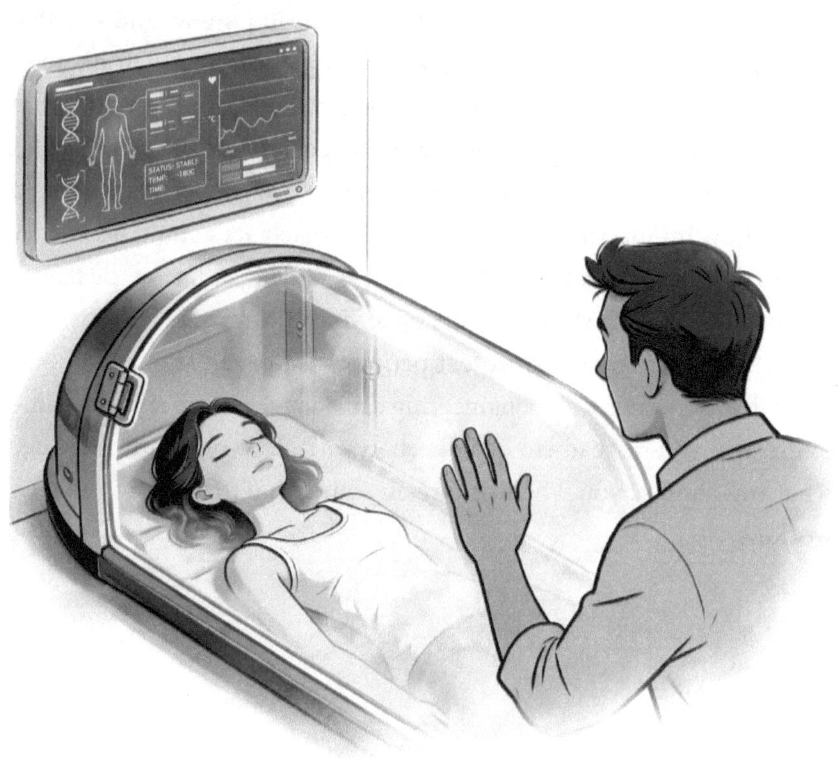
°C
STATUS: STABLE
TEMP: -180C
TIME:

CHAPTER 6

BIOSTASIS

Only one technology available today has a chance of radically extending your life: biostasis. The goal of biostasis is to preserve the structure of your body—especially the brain—immediately after legal death, so that at some point in the future you can be revived. Preservation is accomplished by cold temperatures, chemical fixation, or both.

Biostasis is really the continuation of medical care after modern medicine gives up. Doctors used to quit when the heart stopped, but today we can shock the heart back into action. If someone whose heart stopped in the 19th century could have been put into biostasis and revived today, we would have the technology to start their heart again and treat the underlying cause.

Today, doctors give up when they don't believe a patient can be restored to meaningful health using current technology. That's a reasonable thing to do. But legal death is a prognosis, not a diagnosis, so it's also reasonable to apply biostasis when modern medicine runs out of options. This puts the patient's biology on pause so they have a chance of benefiting from future technology. Ideally, everyone who is failed by modern medicine would have the option to go into biostasis to wait for a cure. That's a massive undertaking, but there's no reason we could not preserve everyone who dies of future-treatable cancer, heart disease, and so on.

There's also precedent in modern medicine. Some surgeries involve cooling down a patient until their heart and brain stop, which gives surgeons more time to perform the operation. As the patient is rewarmed, their heart will start beating again and their brain will reboot. Biostasis is the same idea, but optimized for much longer periods.

While biostasis isn't guaranteed to work, it is scientifically plausible. When your heart stops, most of your cells are still viable. This is why, in a hospital, a quarter of people whose hearts stop can be resuscitated. Biostasis attempts to give people a chance of being revived in the same way. It's true that if your brain is destroyed, you suffer what's called information-theoretic death, with no way back. But as long as the brain's structure is preserved, biostasis beats being buried or cremated—it offers a real chance of revival.

The biostasis motto is: if you're going to die, die in the most reversible way possible.

How to Stop the Clock

Cold temperatures are the most widely used form of biostasis, and the industry that focuses on this approach is called cryonics. To clarify the terminology: cryogenics is the branch of physics and engineering that studies how to produce very low temperatures. Cryopreservation uses those very cold temperatures, together with protective chemicals called cryoprotectants, to store cells, tissues, organs, or whole organisms for long periods. Cryonics is the practice of cryopreserving a person for possible revival when future technology can reverse the preservation process and rejuvenate them to a healthy state. In other words, cryonics patients are cryopreserved using cryogenic technology.

Chemical fixation, on the other hand, uses special chemicals to create bonds between the molecules in tissue. This locks them in place and has been used for over a century to preserve biological specimens. You may have heard of formaldehyde, a chemical that keeps biological samples intact seemingly indefinitely. These chemicals grab onto molecules—mostly proteins—to prevent them from moving, reinforce their structure, and preserve them over time. So where cryonics reduces the rate at which molecules change by lowering their kinetic energy, chemical fixation reduces the rate at which molecules break down by reinforcing them with an atomic scaffold that holds them in place. This process is sometimes referred to as chemopreservation.

Fixed tissue is quite stable, but some organizations that offer chemical fixation also introduce cryoprotectants to allow long-term care at very low temperatures, potentially for hundreds of years. This combination of cryopreservation and chemopreservation is sometimes referred to as vitrifixation.

The main question is whether these methods work for preserving the fine structures of the brain. These include not just the neuronal axons and dendrites that determine which cells are connected, but also the synapses. Synapses are small patches that send and receive chemical signals between neurons and help determine the strength of their connections, so preserving them is crucial to preserving who you are. These fine details of brain structure are sometimes called ultrastructure, and preserving the ultrastructure is currently considered the bar for high-quality biostasis. In laboratory settings, under ideal conditions for preservation, both cryopreservation and chemopreservation have been shown to preserve brain structure. Chemopreservation does this better, but cryopreservation results are also quite good.

In practice, someone would first sign up with a company that provides biostasis services. Typically this would be a cryonics company that does emergency pickup, often with a specialized ambulance. When that person gets sick and is dying, the cryonics company sends a standby team to wait until the customer is declared legally dead. The team then immediately cools the customer down and gives them special medications to protect their brain. The customer is then brought to the company's facility, where they are perfused with a special antifreeze solution called cryoprotectant. This allows the body to be cooled to ultra-low temperature and transition to a glass-like state. Getting someone into this glass-like state is called vitrification. Glass is a solid, so not much changes over time as long as the body is kept cold enough.

While they are vitrified, tiny changes in their body will accumulate due to cosmic rays and other rare events, but, on the whole, they won't change enough for it to make any difference once revived. Their memories and personality won't be altered. The amount of change over

100 years at cryogenic temperatures might be similar to one minute of being alive—nothing to be concerned about.

While no person—or large animal, for that matter—has been vitrified and brought back to life, there are reasons to believe that cryonics will work. First, the same process has been used successfully for decades to store and revive cells, embryos, and tissues. Because of their small size, cells are the easiest to cryopreserve. Some microbes, including bacteria, have been revived after tens of thousands of years in permafrost and ice. Hundreds of thousands of human embryos have been cryopreserved—some for as long as 30 years—and then warmed up, implanted, and born as healthy babies. Animal organs have been vitrified and revived in healthy working order. Even larger structures— such as skin grafts, ovarian tissue, and corneas—have been successfully transplanted after decades in cryogenic storage.

While we don't have proof that an entire animal can safely go to cryogenic temperatures and back, less extreme cold has been shown to be survivable. In 2015, a boy in Missouri fell through ice into a lake. After 15 minutes he was retrieved, but he had no pulse for 45 minutes. Despite this, rescuers revived him and he recovered. Similarly, in 1999 a Swedish radiologist who was skiing in Norway fell into an ice-covered stream. She was trapped under the ice for 80 minutes and her body temperature dropped to 13.7°C. Despite this, a medical team resuscitated her after a few hours.

You may have heard other stories of people who have been trapped in snow avalanches, or fallen into ice-cold water, had their hearts stop beating for over an hour, and yet were later revived without long-term damage. Cases like these have led to sayings among medical practitioners like, "you're not dead until you're warm and dead." In fact, this works so well that doctors sometimes induce hypothermia during critical surgeries involving the heart, lungs, or brain to protect patients.

Don't jump in a frozen river just yet, though. Being in ice water can help preserve you for a few hours, but to last decades you need to be much colder than that. Every 10-degree drop in temperature slows biological time by half, so if you are protected for an hour at 20°C, you'd be protected for years or decades at -120°C. If you go even colder and become vitrified, you should be stable for hundreds or thousands of years.

So while animals and even people in accidents have inadvertently shown the benefits of low temperatures on slowing down metabolism and preventing damage that would have otherwise occurred, cryonics takes this to a whole new level. Patients are cooled to a glass-like state that not only prevents their body from decaying, but is so cold that ice can't form. This means that, in principle, if you can vitrify and rewarm someone properly, they won't change much in between.

This has been proposed as a way for humans to travel to distant stars, but it's also a potential way to travel to the distant future. A future that, hopefully, has advanced medical technology to rewarm you, cure whatever killed you, and rejuvenate your body so you don't die again shortly thereafter.

But nothing as large as a human brain has been vitrified and revived to life. Figuring out how to safely rewarm organs is an area of active research. Fortunately, we don't need to know how to revive people to get them safely into biostasis and, once they are in stasis, we have a lot of time to engineer revival technologies. That's why cryonics companies are more concerned with optimizing the cooling process than the rewarming process. Getting people out of biostasis will happen in the future using future technology, so better now to focus on making sure people have a good experience on the way in.

Factors in Cryopreservation Quality

A good experience means successful vitrification and a safe place to rest. After cryopreservation, patients are kept in a dewar, which is a large metal container filled with liquid nitrogen. They look like oversized stainless-steel water bottles and have the same vacuum-insulated design. In there you can remain cold, stable, and safe.

The trouble is that cooling to and rewarming from extremely low temperatures can be dangerous. These dangers include metabolic damage, ice formation, cracking, dehydration, and toxicity. It's the job of the cryonics company to ensure you make it into and out of biostasis with as little damage as possible, so they spend a lot of time trying to optimize the process.

The number one thing needed for a smooth transition into biostasis is a good starting point. If your brain is relatively healthy and intact, it's easier to preserve than if you have head trauma from a car accident, or if you collapse in the desert and bake under the sun for a few hours.

Starting the preservation process from a healthy state is more complicated than it sounds. Most adults are becoming less healthy over time as aging damage accumulates. The brain structure of a 100-year-old is usually less robust than that of an 80-year-old.

If you were only optimizing the starting condition for biostasis, you would want to enter it as soon as possible, before you accumulate any more damage. However, the trade-off is that the longer you can stay alive, the more biostasis technology will advance. Cryonics technology is improving rapidly, so the benefit to having a healthier brain at the time of vitrification would normally be outweighed by the more advanced technology that could be used later. When it comes to getting started early or doing the hard work of keeping yourself healthy while waiting for new tech, patience is a virtue.

So, for people who have years to live and no signs of neurodegeneration, it's better to wait and see what the biostasis community comes up with. A new innovation might reduce your time in stasis by decades and keep more of your memory intact for when you're revived.

In between those extremes, things are less clear, and you'll have to make your own decision about when to take the cold plunge. In most cases, you will want to stay alive as long as possible.

Everything changes after clinical death. While the brain shrinks and deteriorates gradually throughout life, and this process accelerates in advanced age, the rate of damage accumulation becomes dramatically faster after your heart stops beating. Your cells and tissues are still alive even after your heart stops, but they won't stay viable for long. A day without a heartbeat does more damage than a decade with one.

As soon as blood circulation stops, there's no time to wait—just apply current technology as quickly as possible. For context, you can get a great preservation if you start within a few minutes, or a decent one if you start within a few hours, but things get very bad after a day or two. So there's a huge difference between having a standby team waiting for you at your bedside when you're declared dead and having to wait for them to drive or fly in from another city. Ideally, the preservation would be a planned procedure, which is possible in some states that allow medical aid in dying, where a terminally ill patient can take medication that stops their heart and brain.

So, the best starting point for most people will be a planned procedure far in the future. From there, the number two thing that ensures a good transition into biostasis is perfusion, the process of getting fluids throughout a tissue. Whether you're preserving someone with cold temperatures, chemical fixatives, or both, all methods of biostasis rely on perfusion to protect the patient. This usually means pumping medications and chemicals through the arteries so they can travel throughout the brain and body to protect them.

For vitrification, the fluid contains cryoprotectants that prevent ice crystal formation. If the cryoprotectants don't reach a certain part of the brain in high enough concentration, then that part of the brain will be damaged by ice during the cooling process. For chemical fixation, the fluid contains chemical fixatives that bond molecules. If the fixatives don't reach a certain part of the brain in high enough concentration, then that part of the brain will decay over time. In both cases, a uniform distribution that meets some minimum threshold is ideal.

If people were tiny, this wouldn't be a problem because, for a small tissue sample, introducing chemicals is easy. You can simply immerse it in cryoprotectant or chemical fixative and diffusion will ensure enough gets in there. For something the size of a human organ, immersion would give you good concentrations on the outside, but leave the inside vulnerable. The way around this is to use the vascular system to make the delivery. By pumping the fluid through the vasculature, you get distribution from the inside out. In addition, perfusing cold fluids is the fastest way to lower the patient to safer temperatures.

Another problem with perfusion is that, in most places around the world, you can't start perfusion until after the heart stops beating. Unfortunately, if the flow of blood stops, you can get blood clots and other problems that make it difficult to start circulation again. In this case, perfusing a patient can damage their vasculature and tissues.

However, perfusion injury can be mitigated by adding medications to the infusion that clear blood clots and open blood vessels.

Both cryoprotectant and fixative preservation have some procedural complications due to the size and structure of the human body and brain. Each requires real expertise to perform well so, no matter how tech-savvy you are, don't try this at home.

Once someone is loaded with protective chemicals, the third consideration is how best to cool them down to their long-term storage temperature. With good perfusion, someone who is preserved with chemical fixatives can then be put into a refrigerator to wait for revival, or kept at lower temperatures if cryoprotectant is introduced after initial fixation. For cryonics, the goal is to go much lower—down below the glass transition temperature.

Cooling down to cryogenic temperatures is safer than staying warm, but has some risks that need to be dealt with. Done well, vitrification would leave your tissues in a pristine state. Done poorly, the process damages tissues, and makes it less likely that your brain will be fully recoverable. For example, you can't simply drop someone into a vat of liquid nitrogen and expect them to turn into a nice, glassy statue. Instead, the body would freeze and crack and make it very hard for future doctors to fix you. There are different dangers throughout the entire range of temperatures from human body temperature to liquid nitrogen temperature. Understanding them is the first step to avoiding them.

Dangerous Temperature Ranges

The process of cooling down and warming back up has several danger points. The first is that normal body temperature is healthy when your heart is beating, but unhealthy when it isn't. At body temperature or room temperature, your body will rapidly degrade. If you spend too much time warm without circulation, your own cells will start to damage themselves and their surroundings. So you want to quickly go from body temperature toward the freezing point of water to slow down metabolism. Recall that every 10°C you drop will halve the rate of metabolism, effectively doubling the protection you have.

Below 0°C, metabolism slows way down, but a new danger appears: ice. There are two distinct ice-related problems. The first is ice nucleation, which is where tiny ice crystals start to form. These baby crystals don't do much damage, but they set the stage for the second problem, which is ice-crystal growth. Ice steals the liquid water in your body to grow, which dehydrates cells and tissues. Dehydration can denature proteins, alter concentrations of electrolytes, cause toxicity, and so on. Growing crystals also physically damage surrounding tissue.

The colder you get, the more frequently baby ice crystals form because the relatively slow motion of the molecules makes it easy for them to stick together. Conversely, the warmer you are, the more mobile water is, and the more quickly it finds crystals to freeze to. Modern cryoprotectants are designed to separate the ice nucleation range and ice growth range as much as possible, so they can be dealt with separately. This is safer because when you cool through the relatively warm growth range, no crystals have formed yet and you essentially get to skip one of the danger zones.

The first danger zone is between 0°C and -40°C, which is like winter in northern Canada. If cryoprotectants are present at sufficient concentration for vitrification, then even when you are this cold, you don't have to worry about ice formation. A little metabolic risk remains, so you don't want to spend too much time at these relatively warm temperatures.

The second danger zone is between -40°C and -120°C, which is like winter on Mars. In this range the liquids in your body become exponentially more viscous, until they turn to glass. During this phase, metabolic risk continues to drop exponentially. There's some risk of thermal stress, but the main risk is still ice crystal formation.

The final danger zone is between -120°C and -196°C, which is like a warm day on Jupiter's moon Europa. With modern cryoprotectants, dropping into this range takes you across the glass transition temperature, where your body changes to a solid, glass-like state. Below the glass transition temperature, there's no risk of damage from molecular activity and ice no longer grows.

However, there's a new risk as your temperature continues to drop: fractures. If you take a glass baking dish from a hot oven and pour cold water into it, the dish can break. Similarly, temperature changes during cryopreservation can create cracks that would need to be fixed on revival.

That said, a fracture is in a sense quite orderly. It's easier to reattach a finger that has been cut off than to rebuild one that has been crushed. In the same way, fractures might be relatively easy to repair with future technology.

Once you're at liquid nitrogen temperature, the major risks are unrelated to cryonics itself. You won't deteriorate over time, but you could still get hurt by something like an earthquake.

On the way back up to normal body temperature, the dangers of different temperature ranges are similar but have some new challenges. Starting from liquid nitrogen temperature, warming to the glass-transition temperature involves more risk of cracking. When moving through Europa temperatures, slower is safer.

Once you warm above the glass-transition temperature, ice risk comes back. This is called devitrification and it is where water that was locked in a glass-like state starts rearranging into ice crystals. You can still be far below freezing and yet warm enough for that rearrangement to happen.

There's also the risk of small ice crystals merging into larger ones that do additional damage. Ice crystal growth is more dangerous on the way back up because of the tiny ice crystals that were nucleated on the way down. All those little crystals don't go away when you're vitrified; they just wait around for the chance to grow and wreak havoc. During the rewarming phase, they get enough energy to have their chance. So, during the rewarming process, more ice crystals form, and both old and new crystals grow. This is a case where an ounce of prevention is worth a pound of cure, so cryonics organizations do everything they can to minimize crystal formation during cool-down.

Then, as the temperature rises toward 0°C and you would like to restore biological activity, the cryoprotectant needs to be removed carefully to avoid damage. If you flush out the cryoprotectant too quickly, the dehydrated cells might burst as water rushes in, because water moves through cell membranes faster than the cryoprotectant gets out. Flush it out too slowly and your cells won't be happy when they start running again.

After that, as the temperature passes 0°C and continues to normal body temperature, biological activity can resume. The exponential slowing of metabolism that helped protect you on the way into biostasis now turns into an exponential increase in the rate of metabolism. Pathogens and decomposition reactivate in earnest, accelerated by any damage that was done since the biostasis process started. Of course, repairs would be made before, during, and after rewarming to make sure you emerge in a healthy state. To make repairs as easy as possible, techniques have been developed to minimize the damage that occurs during the preservation process.

Preventing Damage with Cryoprotectants and Controlled Cooling

The two primary techniques for preventing damage during the transition into cryostasis are cryoprotectants and controlled cooling.

As mentioned, cryoprotectants are chemicals that protect the cells and tissues of the body from cold temperatures. They prevent ice crystal formation and growth, like the antifreeze in cars. Controlled cooling allows your body to be cooled slowly through temperature ranges where slow is safe, but rapidly through temperature ranges where it's dangerous. For example, whenever you're in a temperature range where ice crystals are more likely to form or grow, it's best to pick up the pace.

Optimal cooling rates depend on the cryoprotectant formulation and concentration. If you had a perfect cryoprotectant, things would be easy and you could cool at whatever rate you liked. Conversely, the more control you have over cooling rate, the less you need to depend on cryoprotectants.

The main job of modern cryoprotectants is to facilitate vitrification, and they do this by being viscous like oil. This slows down water molecules so they don't have time to join into ice crystals before the body solidifies and stops them from moving entirely. Cryoprotectants help out in other ways as well. One simple way is that when they are added, water comes out of the body, which means less water is available to form ice. Also, just like adding salt to water lowers its freezing point, cryoprotectants make it so that the body can go lower without freezing.

Modern cryoprotectants include ice blockers, which bind to ice crystals to prevent them from growing during cooling and rewarming. This allows them to do a good job of preventing ice-related damage and getting a patient safely into a glass-like state.

Cryoprotectants do more than just slow down ice formation. They are also designed to deal with problems like tissue penetration, toxicity, osmotic stress when water leaves cells, and clogging of the vasculature.

The more cryoprotectant a patient has, the less likely they are to suffer damage from ice. However, as with many things in life, there's a trade-off. High concentrations of cryoprotectant can reduce ice crystal formation, but also lead to higher toxicity for cells. If a cryoprotectant with no toxicity could be found, you could use a lot of it and prevent all ice crystal formation. That would make cryopreservation and revival much easier. Adding additional components can reduce these adverse effects, but nobody has found a cryoprotective cocktail that completely eliminates the downsides.

One way to minimize the damage from cryoprotectant toxicity is to add them to the body after it's relatively cold. Something that is poisonous while your cells are active might not be so bad when they are in slow motion. On rewarming, the cryoprotectant can be removed before the patient gets too warm, further minimizing toxic effects.

Even though these are real problems, they are secondary to ice crystals, not just because these crystals can damage cells and tissues that are being cooled down or warmed up, but also because they cause damage that's hard to repair. It seems likely that cells suffering from dehydration and toxicity will be easier to fix than those that were mangled by ice. Imagine the difference between clearing out some toxic chemicals during rewarming by infusing newer, nontoxic versions, versus trying to do microscopic surgical repairs. So it's a good trade-off to use cryoprotectants now to prevent the worst kinds of damage and shift the burden of things like cryoprotectant toxicity to a time period that's better equipped to handle it.

Modern cryoprotectant mixtures are not perfect, but they have provided a step-function improvement in how easy it should be to revive cryonics patients, and further breakthroughs in cryoprotectants could lead to additional technological jumps. There are research groups doing exciting work designing new cryoprotective agents and, if they succeed, we may see demonstrations of reversible cryostasis in animals soon.

Even with cryoprotectants, there are still some limitations on how well ice formation can be prevented. If your body isn't cooled fast enough, it's possible that ice will form anyway. The critical cooling rate determines the minimum speed of cooling down to avoid ice formation. Similarly, the critical warming rate is how fast you need to warm someone up to avoid forming ice crystals. So anytime you are above the glass transition temperature, if you change temperature too slowly, you give ice crystals more time to form and grow.

Unfortunately, the speed of cooling needs to be balanced with the evenness of cooling throughout the body. If two body areas cool at different rates, you can produce thermal stresses and mechanical damage. The body isn't uniform, which is why it's easy to vitrify a jar of gel but not human bodies. Just as a frozen bottle of water can break its container, the tissues in your body can push on each other as they cool down.

Below the glass transition temperature, these stresses can lead to fractures. This can be mitigated to some extent by cooling patients very slowly. Once you have someone vitrified, you could cool them to liquid nitrogen temperature over the course of months or years to minimize the risk of cracking, but this is difficult in practice, so cracking remains a problem. Until there are methods for rapid, even cooling and rewarming, cryonics will require the heavy use of cryoprotectants.

One concept for cooling much more rapidly is to send cold, inert gas like helium throughout the vasculature. The gas is used after perfusion with cryoprotectants, and creates an internal convective cooling to complement any cooling from the exterior. This technique is called persufflation and it could reduce the need for cryoprotectants because with extremely rapid cooling, ice crystals won't have as much time to form, which means you don't need as much cryoprotectant to slow them down.

Persufflation might also help protect the brain by leaving gas inside the vasculature. This may help prevent cracking because the gas in the vasculature is compressible, essentially leaving small air pockets throughout the glass that make it more like a foam. It also might limit the damage of any fractures that do occur by serving as a barrier to crack propagation.

Another way to use cooling to improve outcomes is to find a temperature that is a sweet spot between ice formation and cracking. Ice growth stops at the glass transition temperature, and the risk of fracturing gets worse from there as temperatures get lower. So dropping from the glass transition temperature to liquid nitrogen temperature is heading into more dangerous territory for cracking. People do it anyway because storing people in liquid nitrogen is much cheaper than keeping them just below the glass transition temperature, and cost is a big factor when you are storing people for potentially very long periods.

To get the benefits of vitrification without fractures, some organizations believe it's safest to remain just below the glass transition temperature. This is called intermediate temperature storage (ITS) and it's being actively tested by cryonics organizations.

The way ITS will work is, instead of using a traditional cryonics dewar, in which a body is immersed in liquid nitrogen, a special ITS dewar is used. In the ITS dewar, a patient's body is kept inside an internal container within the dewar that is surrounded by liquid nitrogen vapor. The internal container has electric heating, which actively maintains the ideal temperature and also keeps it uniform. This approach is more expensive because of the special equipment and power required. It also has the additional risk from power outage. But, if it turns out to have great benefits for reducing damage, it may become the standard approach in cryonics. Vitrification without fractures would probably lead to the most successful and fastest revival, something for which many customers would pay more.

Cryopreservation Versus Chemopreservation

Many of the risks associated with cryonics aren't a concern when it comes to chemical fixation. People who opt for chemopreservation are stored at cold temperatures, but there's no need to lower the temperature so much as to risk fractures. Similarly, the risk of ice crystal formation is zero if the long-term care is at -20°C, the temperature in a standard laboratory freezer, or even a bit lower. The tissues are protected at these relatively warm temperatures by cryoprotectants, and the cryoprotectants give you the option to vitrify later if necessary.

Finally, chemical fixation is currently believed to be the best at preserving information-carrying structures in the brain so, in a revival scenario, you'd come out with more of your memories in mint condition.

With all of these benefits, why would anyone opt for cryopreservation? One reason is that, with our current understanding, it seems easier to revive someone from cryopreservation than to revive them from chemopreservation. First, the toxicity from cryoprotectants could be neutralized, but the toxicity of fixatives cannot. A cryoprotectant might disable a protein by stealing water that the protein needs to maintain its shape, and this could potentially be reversed with advanced medicines, or perhaps not even occur with next-generation cryoprotectants. By contrast, chemical fixatives completely inactivate a protein by bonding to it; it's much more difficult to even imagine how this could be reversed in practice.

Second, revival will probably require the preservation process to be rapidly and evenly reversed. For cryostasis, this means quickly warming someone up, but doing it in a way that's uniform all the way through. It would not be good to have body-temperature skin while your heart and lungs are still cold. This is a hard problem to solve, but people can wrap their heads around the idea of some futuristic sauna that would warm you up safely. It's harder to visualize a method of quickly and uniformly removing chemical cross-links from a big fraction of molecules in every cell, throughout the whole body. So rewarming seems easier than simultaneous chemical cross-link breaking.

To put things into perspective, though, no matter how hard it is to bring someone out of chemical fixation, it's still much easier than, for example, reversing the damage done by straight freezing. Straight freezing means cooling someone to liquid nitrogen temperatures, but without cryoprotectants to reduce ice crystal formation. Without cryoprotectants, ice crystals form and damage cells. Being frozen in this way isn't ideal, but future technology could still theoretically infer the healthy structure of your brain and the rest of the body, if needed, and reconstruct it.

Some people wager that vitrification would be the easiest type of biostasis to reverse, followed by chemical fixation, with straight freezing being the most challenging. However, it's difficult to make predictions, especially about the future. It may turn out that a world with sufficient technology to reverse aging after someone comes out of cryopreservation is also advanced enough to reverse chemical cross-links. Or perhaps only a few decades are required to go from one to the next, which is faster than a blink of an eye for someone in biostasis. It's even possible that the starting point of a chemically fixed brain will turn out to be easier to repair for some reason, and people who choose chemical fixation will be revived first.

While it's useful to compare and contrast how different biostasis techniques work in theory, there are real-world considerations that matter as well. For example, most of the scientific and industrial effort in biostasis is currently going into cryonics, so cryonics companies are larger and serve wider areas.

Perhaps because of this popularity, much more of the research in biostasis is around how to make the cryopreservation process safer and more effective. So even if you think chemical fixation is a superior technological strategy, in practice you might still want to opt for the more popular approach to benefit from network effects and existing infrastructure.

Network effects are important for another reason. One thing that both camps agree on is that it's valuable to enter biostasis as quickly as possible to limit metabolic damage. Regardless of which process is theoretically superior under laboratory conditions, it's probably preferable to sign up for the one that will be readily available to you when you need it.

Because of this, if you compare current offerings on the market, the cryonics that's available for purchase right now is safer for most people than the chemical-fixation alternatives that exist today. The infrastructure and organizations around cryonics have a significant head start, wider coverage areas, and more capacity to respond to emergencies.

There are also practical reasons to prefer chemical fixation. For example, cryonics can be very expensive whereas chemical fixation can be much cheaper. If someone is interested in biostasis but can't afford a cryonics membership, they should consider the chemical-fixation route. Chemopreserved patients also need less attention and maintenance, so choosing it could help in scenarios where supply lines are disrupted.

For those who can't decide, there's always the option to do both with vitrifixation. Sometimes called aldehyde-stabilized cryopreservation, this adds to the complexity of the procedure, but this combination might lead to the most stable biostasis currently possible. If so, it could be the safest choice, though options for this approach are currently limited. Vitrifixation typically means first applying fixation—with a focus on the brain—followed by introducing cryoprotectants to allow for vitrification. Then the brain can be taken down to cryogenic temperatures. If the brain is both fixed and cryopreserved, and then kept in a solid, glassy state, its structure should remain the most stable over time, potentially for thousands of years.

So the current strategies for biostasis are cryonics, fixation, or vitrifixation. Each has advantages and disadvantages, and many factors that affect how well preserved you are likely to be. However, because operations can have a bigger impact on preservation quality than technology, it's important to know the basics of biostasis operations.

The Real-World Preservation Process

Despite the technical challenges, modern biostasis techniques have been shown to do quite a good job preserving the brain, assuming the procedure is done in a timely and effective manner. However, not all procedures take place under ideal conditions. Logistical and operational factors still come into play in real-world cases.

Field teams who are trying to get a human body into biostasis have to deal with regulatory constraints, hospital rules and regulations, traffic, the logistics of moving the team and the chemicals across distances, and myriad other challenges. Because real-world complexities can impact the effectiveness of a biostasis procedure, you'll be in the best position to take advantage of biostasis, and contribute to this most important industry, if you have a detailed understanding of how a cryonics case happens in practice.

If you find yourself warming to the idea of cryonics, the first step is to sign up with a company or nonprofit institution that performs cryopreservation. Get the people you care about signed up too, so you don't end up scrambling to arrange cryopreservation in the heat of the moment.

As part of onboarding, you would let the provider know where you live and some other basic information. You may need to start paying a monthly membership fee and also sign up for a life insurance policy that would cover the costs of cryopreservation upon your untimely demise. With the financing all set up, you would then tell your friends and family about your wishes and ask them to please, please, please make sure the cryonics organization knows if you ever get seriously ill or injured.

Usually, you would live a nice long life and end up dying slowly of some age-related condition. Suppose you come down with an incurable cancer and you only have a few weeks to live. If your arrangements are with a cryonics organization, at this point they would need to be informed to begin preparations. They might then send a team—sometimes in an ambulance full of special equipment—to your location and that team would wait for the sad news.

The team would then follow a three-step process of standby, stabilization, and transport. The goal of this process is to keep the brain as healthy as possible by contemporary biological criteria. This minimizes the amount of damage that can accumulate before you enter biostasis.

During the standby phase, the team prepares their equipment and then just hangs out. If allowed, they will stay in or near the room where you're dying, waiting for a doctor or nurse to declare you legally dead. Once you're legally dead, the team immediately jumps into action to stabilize you.

The goal of stabilization is to prevent the rapid decline that would otherwise take place after your heart stops. In other words, to keep your brain in the best possible shape until cryoprotectants can be introduced. When the standby team takes possession of your barely dead body, even though you no longer have brain activity, your brain cells don't all die immediately. So in some sense you are still alive, and the standby team will treat you that way. They don't want to resuscitate you, but they do everything else to keep you healthy.

Keeping your brain cells happy is paramount, and doing that well requires keeping your arteries and veins in working order. An unhealthy or dying vasculature is more likely to block up or rupture, which prevents fluids from getting to where they need to be. This is called ischemia, and it's the major operational challenge in the field.

To prevent this, the stabilization process involves using cardiopulmonary support, cooling, and medications. Circulation is usually maintained with chest compressions at first, and later with a perfusion machine. Cardiopulmonary support aims to supply your cells with oxygen and nutrients so they don't realize anything is out of the ordinary. It also helps to cool you down, and the lower the temperature, the less oxygen and nutrients are needed. Circulatory support keeps the vasculature open so that medications, organ preservation solution, and eventually cryoprotectants can be perfused throughout the body, the last being critical for successful vitrification.

To cool you down, you would be placed in an ice bath. The ice-cold water would be continuously recirculated over your body to increase the cooling rate. Hypothermia is one of the most effective ways to keep cells viable, so the faster the team can get you just above freezing, the better.

The fastest way to cool you, though, is to circulate cold fluid through your vasculature. At some point in the process, the cryonics team will hook up a pump to your arteries and veins that can circulate cold organ preservation solution and then cryoprotectant through the body.

Many cryonics organizations will introduce a variety of medications as they cool down the body. The aim is to protect your cells and tissues even beyond what circulation and low temperatures can do. The cocktail of medications includes things like anticoagulants to prevent clots from clogging up your vasculature, thrombolytics to clear any clots that already formed, neuroprotectants to defend the brain, drugs to help prevent brain swelling, pH buffers to neutralize acidification, as well as vasopressors to maintain pressure in the blood vessels. The team may also use other ingredients they think will help, like antioxidants and anti-inflammatory medications.

One of the most important medications has the dual role of protecting your brain and ensuring that you remain fully unconscious.

This is necessary because there's a small risk that circulating oxygenated blood could cause someone to wake up the same way that performing CPR sometimes wakes up a person whose heart has stopped.

Some cryonics organizations use ambulances where your blood would be washed out and replaced with an organ preservation solution to prevent clotting, in the hope of keeping the vasculature functioning. The solution is isotonic, nutritious, and cold.

Then you would be perfused with cryoprotectant. Cryoprotectant is crucial for safely descending to cryogenic temperatures, so this process is critical. The cryoprotectant needs to reach the correct concentration to be effective, but it needs to be introduced slowly. The most effective way to deliver cryoprotectants throughout the brain is through the circulatory system; that's why so much time is spent up front making sure the vasculature remains functional.

One difficult part of achieving high cryoprotectant concentrations in the brain is that the blood-brain barrier, which is good at preventing bad stuff from getting into your brain, is also good at preventing cryoprotective agents from getting in. Unfortunately, this is just the place where they are needed the most. Fortunately, modern cryoprotectants have components that are fairly good at crossing the blood-brain barrier, so vitrification is still achievable.

As cryoprotectant is added to your body, the team will also continue to cool you down to about 0°C, to help further reduce metabolic damage, but also to avoid any potential toxicity from the high concentrations of the cryoprotectant itself. Your temperature and the concentration of cryoprotectant will be monitored throughout the process until sufficient levels are reached.

Then your body would be prepared for the third phase: transport. The goal of transport is to make sure your body gets to a long-term storage facility safely and quickly. The team needs to keep you cold during transit to minimize molecular damage. Even at near-freezing temperatures, the enzymes and other molecules in your body are still active, just at a slower rate. That's why you need to get cooled down even more later, and why there's a rush to get you to the cryonics facility in a reasonable time.

To keep you cool, you might be sealed in an insulated container filled with dry ice. You will then be driven or flown to the long-term storage facility. Once there, you can be taken through the final stages, using specialized equipment with better temperature control over longer periods of time.

When you arrive at the facility, you'll be put into a cooling chamber where you can be cooled, eventually to the glass transition temperature to get you to a vitrified state. While in the chamber, you'll be sprayed with liquid nitrogen to rapidly cool you to around -100°C. Then cooling is paused to allow the temperature throughout your body to equalize. After that, cooling can start again either to an intermediate temperature just below the glass transition temperature or to liquid nitrogen temperature. To prevent cracking due to thermal stresses, the cooling sequence is: fast, pause, slow, stop.

Once you're at the long-term care temperature, the best biostasis organizations currently in operation would use CT scans to evaluate the structure of the brain, to see how much cryoprotectant was delivered to each part of the brain, and if any ice was formed.

No vitrification is perfect, but some companies today can demonstrate that the concentrations of cryoprotectant sufficient to vitrify were delivered to most regions of the brain, and this can be clearly seen on CT scans of the head. You might see some imperfect delivery to the skin or fat, but the brain often looks good from this standpoint. For those who opt in, some companies may also take a small sample of neural tissue from either a nonessential part of the brain or the spinal cord. This is then used for electron microscopy to see the preservation quality of the ultrastructure—the very tiny details of the neurons. This test is the current state of the art for how well the preservation was done, and you should prefer companies that use this feedback mechanism to improve their processes.

After quality control, you will be moved to a dewar. Dewars are designed to be easy to maintain—someone simply needs to occasionally pour a little liquid nitrogen in to account for any that has evaporated. The dewar is then monitored for temperature, liquid nitrogen levels, and any signs of needing to be replaced.

Once in your dewar, you can just sit back, relax, and wait for science and technology to catch up with you.

Improving Operations

Fortunately, keeping the site secure and topping off the liquid nitrogen in your container to compensate for whatever evaporated is most of the work of maintaining a cryonics facility. Liquid nitrogen is cheap, and one person could look after thousands of patients, so the economics are feasible. Over the course of decades a lot can change, so you'll want to pick a cryonics organization that has plans, backup plans, and fail-safes for many different situations. Not only that, but also a desire to get better every year.

Speaking of which, there are many ways to improve existing procedures. The simplest would be to have a hospice care facility located next to the long-term storage facility. Then, if you're diagnosed with a terminal disease, you can go to the location where your cryonics organization does the preservation process. If you're diagnosed with a terminal condition that will destroy your brain, then you may need to both relocate and end your life voluntarily. Here, having favorable laws around medical aid in dying, which is physician-assisted death, becomes important. There's an option of VSED, which stands for voluntary stopping of eating and drinking, but this end-of-life option is much worse, so talk to your doctor before considering it.

Better assisted death laws would help in almost every biostasis case, because teams would not need to wait for the patient to be declared dead. Once legal death is imminent, they could take over cardiopulmonary support and administer drugs to help the patient pass peacefully, while giving the best possible protection to their brain and cardiovascular system. Some biostasis organizations only accept patients via medical aid in dying to ensure they provide the best possible preservation. It may seem strange that people with a desire to live forever would want to end their life quickly, but when you have a terminal condition, biostasis is the one longevity therapy worth dying for.

In the meantime, the best thing you can do to ensure good preservation quality is to minimize the delay between legal death and the biostasis team starting their procedure. For example, you could make sure that you're under the care of a biostasis-friendly doctor who can immediately declare legal death. Or that you're in a hospice facility where a 24/7 nursing staff can declare legal death.

Some risks are less about individual circumstances and more about the industry. There's risk that the organization looking after you will fall apart. There's a risk that a hurricane or other natural disaster could physically destroy you, your dewar, or the facility that you're in. There's risk of political upheaval; for instance some people who don't like the idea of biostasis might decide to attack the facility and wreck everything.

All of these risks and more have been considered by biostasis providers. Unfortunately, there's no perfect solution that will guarantee your safety while in biostasis, just like there's no way to guarantee your safety while alive. However, in both cases things can be done to greatly reduce the risk to you.

The biggest way to reduce risk is for cryonics to become as big as possible. Economies of scale will make it much cheaper to provide the service, much more common, and much more socially acceptable. The more people there are in biostasis, the more people there are who will have some friend or relative in this state, waiting to be brought back. With societal approval, strong economics, and the incentives of many people aligned with biostasis, those in biostasis will have the best odds of coming out of it alive.

The rate at which biostasis could grow is more limited by demand than technology. You could get everyone who dies each year into biostasis for a few billion dollars by building large facilities. Think of huge, insulated, underground tanks with small openings on top. Similar storage tanks have already been built to house natural gas, and the process would only require a small percentage of the world's production of liquid nitrogen or chemical fixatives. A few billion dollars may seem like a lot of money, but there are people who could personally finance that kind of operation, let alone companies or other large organizations.

Besides scale, there are other strategies for protecting patients. One is organizational structure. By separating the organizations that perform preservation, those responsible for long-term care, and those that do research, it's possible to keep each in check. By selecting long-term care locations that are in places with political and geological stability, other risks can be mitigated as well. By continuing to develop biostasis technology, those who are trying to help biostasis patients will be empowered to keep them in the best shape possible, and revive them as soon as possible.

Improving Technology

While there are many ways to improve the operational, legal, and social aspects of biostasis, the resources needed to really do a good job with those may depend on continued progress on the technology side. Seeing is believing, so the biggest boost to biostasis might be a demonstration of revival in a mammal, like a mouse. If a mouse can be vitrified and then rewarmed to live out a normal, healthy life, cryonics will probably get the support it needs to become a common, if not the most common, choice at the end of life.

Technology to cryopreserve and revive a mouse is far from what would be needed for a human, but seeing a cute little critter walking around after going through the process could inspire many people to give biostasis a try.

Technological progress is needed for more immediate concerns as well. While the preservation quality already being achieved under ideal conditions seems sufficient for revival, continued advances could lead to additional benefits such as high quality preservation under a wider variety of circumstances and shorter time to revival. Any advances in protocols, equipment, perfusion techniques, cryoprotectants, fixatives, and cooling strategies could help more people get safely into biostasis and, hopefully, more people successfully come out of it.

For cryonics to work better, in particular, the biggest technological opportunity is improving cryoprotectants. To do a good job, a cryoprotectant must be able to get to all the places it needs to go, and in high enough concentration. To get a cryoprotectant to the right location, you want one that has good penetration and low viscosity. To get the right concentration, you want a low minimum concentration for vitrification.

The ideal cryoprotectant we are pursuing is unfreezable, minimally viscous, permeable, and nontoxic. Unfreezable is to prevent ice damage. Minimal viscosity helps it spread throughout the body. Permeability helps it get into cells and prevent dehydration damage. Nontoxicity helps keep cells viable. That's quite a few competing priorities, which is one reason current cryoprotectants are good, but not perfect.

Modern cryoprotectants contain vitrification agents like ethylene glycol, ice blockers with names like Z-1000, and a few other things. Everything except the active cryoprotective agents is called the carrier solution. All of the ingredients work together to minimize the damage done by both the vitrification process and the cryoprotectant itself.

Ice blockers help by preventing the growth of ice crystals. They can block ice from crystallizing along a plane, like a sheet of ice on a pond. Naturally occurring ice blockers in fish work this way, and help them survive in ice-cold water. Wood frogs freeze in the winter only to start swimming again in spring. Ice blockers can also prevent water from crystallizing into spikes. Some insects have ice blockers that work in this manner, and the Antarctic midge used them to become the only native insect to that continent. Both types of ice blockers reduce our reliance on cryoprotectants, which helps with both toxicity and viscosity.

We can take inspiration from animals that naturally produce cryoprotectants in many ways. First, by learning from the structure of the molecules that help them survive freezing conditions, we can copy them and make new, improved versions. Second, we might be able to adapt their strategy of having ice blockers available throughout the body on demand. For example, we might be able to create a gene therapy that produces cryoprotectant inside cells whenever the body cools below a certain temperature. Additionally, you could have the same therapy produce enzymes that neutralize the cryoprotectant at higher temperatures. Thus, your body could be prepared for cryonics well ahead of any emergency.

Another technique that deserves more investigation for cryopreservation is annealing. This means holding the temperature steady or gently varying it for a period of time to allow the internal stresses caused by temperature gradients to relax.

We'll want to continue to improve fixation technologies as well. Ever since the 1890s, scientists have been able to preserve brains with fixatives, and newer fixatives like glutaraldehyde have been shown to preserve the microscopic structures of the brain. However, these results were achieved under laboratory conditions. Ensuring that fixatives can be perfused throughout the brain successfully in emergency situations could lead to cheap, widely available, and high-confidence chemopreservation.

Improved perfusion is important for both fixation and cryonics. No matter how good your fixative, or how powerful your cryoprotectant, it will lead to disappointing results if it can't reach every part of your brain. More testing of delivery routes, perfusion parameters, and ways of crossing the blood-brain barrier is needed.

Improvements could also be made in the technology to assess how well the preservation process is going in real time, rather than merely checking the results after the fact. Ideally you would want ways to measure perfusion during the process to allow providers to adapt and adjust. Currently, you can measure the liquid that comes out of the veins to check how much water or cryoprotectant is being absorbed or released by the brain—but can we do better?

You could also use a CT scanner to check how well-perfused the brain is during the perfusion process, just like checking how well the brain was preserved after vitrification. For a more invasive view, you could cut a hole in the skull and actually watch the brain directly. This may sound drastic, but it has proved to be a useful technique for catching things like brain swelling.

Another way to improve outcomes is to simplify the problem. The smaller something is, the easier it is to preserve and revive. While the brain is much smaller than the body, it contains the most important parts of who you are. So focusing primarily on brain preservation and revival will help speed things along. It may be possible to simplify things even more as we gain a deeper understanding of how the brain works and which parts are essential for personality and which are generic and replaceable.

Another potential tailwind is better understanding the practical threshold for successful preservation. We lose brain cells every year in adulthood, so losing a few while in stasis might not be a big problem. The question is how well you need to preserve your brain to make biostasis worth your while. It's known that organs can withstand some amount of ice formation and still function after rewarming. The brain is no exception, and it may be that imperfect preservation still leads to strong memory recall, equivalent personality traits, and good quality of life after revival. If the memory loss after revival is similar to what would happen naturally over a few years, then reinforcing your memories with a journal or a time capsule might help you recover most of what is forgotten.

While good preservation is and should remain the primary focus of biostasis organizations, it also makes sense to spend some time on the technology that might ultimately be used for revival as well as the operational procedures we use today that could make revival easier in the future.

Revival

The goal of biostasis is to eventually revive those who enter it. That means being repaired, warmed back up, and brought back to consciousness. Repair must include fixing up any damage that occurred from entering and leaving biostasis, as well as any age-related damage, illness, or trauma that a person may have had beforehand.

For cryonics patients, rewarming needs to be rapid and even to prevent additional ice crystal formation. This requires controlled delivery of energy throughout the body. For example, a large machine might blast your body with sound waves to warm it up quickly and evenly. After you're warm, medical teams would start intensive care and life support protocols. Once your body is barely dead again, they would apply future medical technology to cure diseases, boost your immune system, rejuvenate your skin, muscle, and bones, and so on.

The specifics of what would be needed will depend on each patient's preservation quality and previous illness. If you died of heart failure and had a stunning cryopreservation, then revival might simply mean warming you back up and doing a heart transplant. If you had some plaque buildup in your arteries, it might make sense to remove those while you're still cold. Other types of damage might be amenable to repair at cold temperatures as well.

If you had more widespread damage from trauma or metastatic cancer, then more work would be needed to fix you up before bringing you back to consciousness. We don't know exactly how the process will work. The truth is, we don't even know if it will work. This whole notion of relying on technological progress in the future may seem a little vague and fanciful. However, there has been quite a bit of technological progress over the last century, so it's not out of the realm of possibility that the people 100 years from now will be able to build a device to warm you and put you back to working order, just as today's technology could repair a broken hip that seemed irreparable 100 years ago.

One reason to be optimistic for cryostasis revival is that current technology can already rewarm small organs. For example, a rat kidney was successfully vitrified, rewarmed, and transplanted into an animal. There are unpublished reports that pig kidneys work after vitrification as well.

So little time and money has gone into exploring revival that it's possible we already have the technological sophistication to do it, but we just don't know it yet. Unfortunately, lack of time and attention has prevented us from exploring the boundaries of what is currently possible. Even if human revival isn't achievable today, biostasis allows us to wait for future opportunities.

We don't have to completely leave the harder problems for the future, though. Adjusting the way we cryopreserve patients today could potentially make it much easier to control the rewarming process. For example, we could introduce additives into the medications that are perfused into patients to make rewarming easier. One additive under investigation is nanoparticles that can be vibrated with magnetic fields. If your tissue contains these nanoparticles, then anyone who tries to rewarm you can use a magnetic field to generate microscopic motion in those particles to heat up the surrounding tissue.

Without nanoparticles, there are still other options like dielectric rewarming, electromagnetic radiation, and ultrasound. These are the main rewarming techniques currently under investigation, but who knows what engineers will dream up while you're taking the long, cold nap.

More reason for hope is that unfreezing technologies seem possible with today's technology. The goal is to quickly and evenly rewarm a block of heterogeneous tissue. An electric blanket won't do it, but more sophisticated energy transfer devices could. For example, machines that use arrays of sound beams to transfer energy appropriately throughout the volume of your brain are being tested. The first version might not work well enough to revive someone without causing damage, but the first rocket didn't reach the moon either.

Biological revival from chemopreservation is a very different challenge. The reversal of chemical fixation involves breaking large numbers of chemical bonds throughout every cell and tissue in the body. Like rewarming, this needs to be done rapidly and evenly so that some parts aren't metabolically active while others are still in stasis. It's currently believed that this will be a much harder problem to solve than rewarming. So if reversing vitrification takes decades to centuries, reversal of chemical fixation might take centuries to millennia. All the same, those planning to go the route of chemical fixation can rest easy knowing that the process very efficiently preserves the structure of their brain.

Once biostasis is shown to be reversible, it will have achieved what is known as suspended animation, where there are no downsides to pausing your biology. Healthy people could use biostasis for long space trips. Sick people could be suspended until doctors or medications are ready to heal them. Biostasis works regardless of what ails you, so ideally anyone who wanted to put their suffering on pause while they wait for a cure could do so. You only live once but, with biostasis, it's okay to take a break once in a while.

Nobody goes into preservation perfectly healthy and, even if they did, no preservation is perfect. So everyone will need some sort of repair. For many people, repair of the body will probably mean simply replacing it with a new one, but repair of the brain is a more complex problem. So, it's useful to speculate on what a hypothetical brain reconstruction might look like to guide decisions about what types of damage to focus on, what types of experiments to pursue, and so on.

Suppose your brain is cryopreserved, but not perfectly. You get some low level of ice crystal formation and some amount of toxicity due to cryoprotectants, but no fractures. What might the doctors of the future do?

One option might be to take some of your cells, grow lots of them, and turn them into all the different cell types they might need for reviving you. Then use those cells to grow new organs and tissues. Next, robots operate on your brain at cryogenic temperature. They clear out the vasculature, adding new vitrified cells and ECM where needed. The brain is then rapidly and evenly rewarmed, perhaps with ultrasound or electromagnetic radiation. As the brain is warming, it becomes possible to perfuse it again. So, perfusion can be used to help with rewarming but also repair. For example, you might perfuse the latest generation of nontoxic cryoprotectants to replace the older versions.

As your brain gets even warmer, all cryoprotectant would be removed and replaced with fluids to support cell health, and then those would be replaced with blood. The brain is then connected to a life support device that provides oxygen, nutrition, temperature control, physical support, medication, sensory input, and output reading—whatever the brain needs to be healthy. Any diseases that were previously untreatable would be treated, including age-related damage.

Once your brain is confirmed to be healthy, it would be transplanted into your new body. After waking up, you would go through a period of physical therapy where you learn to use your new arms, legs, and so on. Then you could catch up on all the technological development, history, and entertainment you missed. Oh, and you'll need to check all your missed messages...

Personal Strategy

Now you know a good deal about biostasis, and the question is how to best incorporate it into your own plan for radical life extension. Given the lack of other options currently available, it makes sense for most people to sign up for biostasis and support the biostasis community. You should familiarize yourself with the various biostasis providers and services on the market, decide which is best for you, and sign up for a plan.

While this should make you feel safer, you shouldn't take your biostasis membership as a license to take up extreme sports. With how rapidly the technology is improving recently, it makes sense to try to stay alive and healthy as long as possible to benefit from any near-term advances.

You should make sure that your friends and family understand your desire to be put into biostasis, as families can be a big help when they understand your wishes, but can also interfere with the process when they don't. Some families have even tried to prevent cryopreservation to get the insurance money that was set aside to pay for it, so be careful.

Also, ensure that your living situation makes it easy for biostasis response teams to get to you as rapidly as possible. For instance, don't live alone in a remote area. It's stressful enough for the standby teams, who are taking your life into their hands—don't make it any harder than it needs to be. Consider moving to a jurisdiction that allows for physician-assisted death to make your cryopreservation a planned procedure. And make sure that if you suddenly keel over, someone will find out about it quickly. It doesn't matter how close you are to a cryonics facility if nobody is checking in on you periodically.

Hopefully, you won't need to go through the actual cryopreservation process because longevity technology will advance fast enough for you to reach longevity escape velocity. That said, hope for the best, but plan for the worst. If you find revival plausible then—absent any proven alternative—it's among the few concrete steps available. For the same reasons, contributing to the biostasis field might be a valuable use of your time.

You should also consider the risks of neurodegeneration and plan around them. If you acquire certain neurodegenerative diseases, then every year you remain out of biostasis, the more damage your brain suffers and the greater your risk of disaster. Disaster could mean the slow degeneration of your brain that ultimately makes it meaningless to go into biostasis. Or, it could mean losing agency and ending up in a situation where your desire to be cryopreserved isn't honored. Either way, you would have been better off taking the cold plunge sooner rather than later.

On the other hand, for someone who is in relatively good health, the progress made in cryonics technology while you're aging outweighs the risk of being out and about. It would be a shame to be put into biostasis a few years before a big breakthrough that helps not only preserve your memories and personality in higher fidelity, but also shortens the duration that you're in biostasis. Of course, you must evaluate the different risks for yourself but, for many people, it will be preferable to hold off on biostasis until there's an urgent medical reason to embrace it.

Holding off has another benefit as well. While you're active, you have the opportunity to influence the course of events. You can dedicate your time and resources into improving the technology, community, and culture around biostasis. You can help protect yourself and others by making biostasis more mainstream and more widely used. You can help save more people by encouraging them to sign up, which will allow efficiencies of scale to bring the costs down—saving even more lives. There are plenty of reasons to remain an active player in this space as long as you can.

One other thing to consider is your own philosophy around survival. Do you insist on having a biological body, or would you be okay having your biological brain in a robotic body? Do you insist on repairing your original brain, or would an exact biological copy be good enough? Do you want a biological brain, or would you be okay with your brain being emulated on a computer? Many revival strategies are possible, and each has different implications for which technology to choose, how long you will be in biostasis and what life will be like after revival. So your personal philosophy and preferences should be made clear to help guide your caretakers.

Just to recap, what would an ideal path to biostasis look like today? You would keep your brain and vasculature healthy throughout your life with lifestyle interventions. You would move close to a preservation facility located in a region that allows assisted suicide. When you're terminally ill, you should go to the facility before aging or disease causes too much damage to your brain and vasculature. You could have a see-you-soon party with your friends or family.

The party may seem frivolous, but at least consider spending a little time with people you care about. Maybe go out to dinner one last time. Give your kids or grandchildren something for safe-keeping.

Afterwards, you'd go to a pre-operating room and lie down on a comfortable bed. They'd play your favorite song and give you medications to make you sleep.

Next the team would perform some preparatory procedures, like establishing access to your circulatory system. Since you're still alive and functioning, they can take their time and make sure everything is perfect. Then the team would take you through physician-assisted death that would maximize your chances of being well preserved.

The process would transition you smoothly from being legally alive to being legally dead with minimal interruption to the flow of nutrients and oxygen to your tissues. Life support systems would keep blood oxygenated and flowing while medications are introduced and temperature is reduced. Dedicated machines would perfuse the right medications at the right time, eventually replacing your blood entirely with protective fluids.

Then you would be seamlessly transitioned into a rapid cooling machine that would take you down to temperatures where all the molecules in your body stop moving. You would be scanned and tested to make sure everything turned out well.

Your team would continue cooling you to your long-term storage temperature. You would be scanned for quality checking, then moved into a dewar, where your neighbors are guaranteed not to be too noisy.

For everyone else, time marches slowly on. But for you, you will either never wake up, or you will wake up immediately in a new world— the same comfortable bed, the same music playing, and, hopefully, many of the same people waiting to welcome you back.

Key Takeaways

Biostasis has not been proven to work for large animals, so there's a wide range of opinions about how plausible it is that someone going into biostasis today could be revived at some point in the future. Currently there are no known reasons why it could not work but that's no guarantee. However, it seems likely that fortune favors the cold. You should make your own decision about how likely you think cryonics or chemopreservation are to work when making plans for your own path to radical life extension.

However, if someone you care about is going to die in the next 10 years, this is probably their best option. Just to be crystal clear, there's only one potential solution to aging right now and it's biostasis. Furthermore, we don't know when we will get a better option. Fortunately, biostasis seems to be working reasonably well, and there's a lot of low-hanging fruit. So even if your time horizon is short, you could still have a big impact by investing or working in biostasis.

Until you're at the end of life, consider ways you can help improve preservation compounds and their delivery. Any advance in either category could lead to big changes in how long it takes for you and others to be revived. If you have an engineering, medical, or scientific background, get involved in technological development. Or, if you have the resources, donate to research efforts. The number of organizations currently working in cryonics research is quite small, so a relatively small amount of money would make a huge difference.

If nothing else, get as many people signed up as possible. Especially if they are near the end of life, discuss biostasis with them. More people means more support from members as well as their friends and family. Not to mention that every new biostasis contract is a chance to save a life.

There's a long to-do list, and the biostasis community needs help with it. Ideas need to be fleshed out, prototyped, tested, and, ideally, built into businesses that can then integrate with the existing industry. Opportunities to improve the biostasis industry abound, and these are just the tip of the iceberg.

So let's not give up on people just because modern medicine can't help them. Future technology might be able to, so we should continue to care for people the best we can if that's their wish. Keep people healthy until disease or aging makes it impossible to keep them alive, and then put them into biostasis. Maybe one day every hospital will have a biostasis team on standby, and everyone will have the option.

Today biostasis is speculative, but that won't be the case forever. At some point improvements in technology will demonstrate that revival is possible. Later it will become routine. Future biostasis technology will preserve you so well that your metabolic arrest might only last a short time. As technology progresses, people who entered biostasis earlier and earlier will become revivable. Eventually, we'll fix everyone who has been waiting and biostasis will only be for short-term storage in the case of emergencies, space voyages, and so on. This period of restoration will be exciting, like opening a million time capsules. People will be reunited with their loved ones, and they'll get to live again.

Cryonics is the first real hope that humans have of achieving radically longer lifespans. It's a way to pause biology until the technology improves enough to cure diseases and reverse aging. Some say the odds are low, but are your best odds located inside a dewar, coffin, or urn?

Consider biostasis to be the foundation of your strategy for radical life extension. Many people think of biostasis as plan B, but what is plan A? They don't have one. For radical life extension, cryonics is plan A and, if you aren't happy about that, you should be pushing with everything you have to build an alternative.

We don't know what that alternative will be, but there is one strategy that seems most likely to keep you from needing biostasis in the first place: therapeutic replacement.

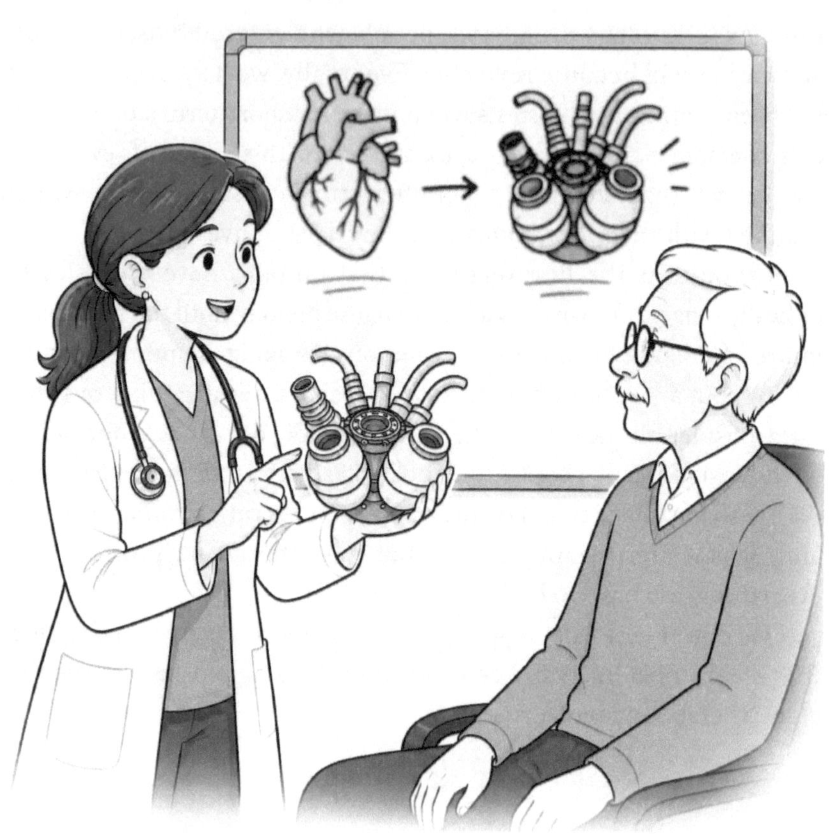

CHAPTER 7

REPLACEMENT

Replacement is the fastest and surest way to defeat aging. Replacement therapies substitute healthy body components for ones that are diseased, damaged, or lost. This medical strategy has a long history of success, encompassing treatments such as blood transfusions, artificial joints, and organ transplants, among others. Its viability stems from a straightforward yet profound principle: replacing damaged components is often easier and more effective than attempting to cure diseases through drug development.

Replacement is powerful for another reason. Recovery of normal function using replacement doesn't require disease mechanisms to be completely characterized, nor does it require new drugs to be developed. Instead, it circumvents the need to engage diseases at a molecular level, and can thus offer a shorter path to the clinic, attractive risk profiles, and solutions for otherwise poorly understood problems like aging. Furthermore, a particular replacement therapy doesn't cure a single disease—it cures every disease in whatever is replaced. It doesn't matter if a patch of your skin is burned, infected, cancerous, or all three. If a surgeon swaps in new skin, any and all of those problems go away.

That's why when some unknown disease is causing pulmonary fibrosis that destroys your lungs, only replacement can help you. Even in situations where the underlying mechanism is understood, like when viral hepatitis ruins someone's liver, sometimes there is no medicine that can cure it. Again, the only option is replacement. And the condition that's probably least understood, and that certainly lacks effective treatments, is aging.

So, why aren't we extensively using replacement to cure diseases and reverse aging? The core problem is supply. Currently, replacement organs come almost exclusively from donors, and this system is so limited that even people in dire need sit on waiting lists for months or years to get just one. Donor organs are precious resources that are reserved for those who fall into a narrow range between desperately sick and hopeless. However, you can imagine that if we had an unlimited supply of organs, then everybody who needed them could get them on demand. If you had an endless source of kidneys, then we would not limit their use to people with stage 5 chronic kidney disease; we'd also give them to people with stage 4 so they never get to stage 5. But why stop there? Maybe people with stage 3 would like some too. The whole calculus flips: when you no longer have to ration organs, medicine shifts from reactive to proactive.

In the same way, if supply were unlimited, it would make sense to give young tissues and organs to old but otherwise healthy people. They might be relatively healthy for their age at the moment, but we know for certain that something is going to break soon. It could be safer to risk a surgery while they are relatively healthy than to try to fix things up after they have had a heart attack, aneurysm, or similar.

Replacement in Current Clinical Practice

While replacement to reverse aging is a future prospect, we aren't starting from zero. Replacement is already in widespread use to treat disease and has been so successful that it has been applied throughout the entire body. In current clinical practice, replacement happens at many levels.

At the smallest scale, simple molecules can be replaced to treat conditions where the body can't produce them. For example, people who can't make certain digestive enzymes can be given pills full of enzymes that help restore their digestive function. Other kinds of enzyme replacement therapy can be administered intravenously to help with so-called storage diseases, where cells don't produce the enzymes necessary to break down certain lipids, sugars, or other molecules, and these substances accumulate—are stored—in the cells.

Similarly, hormone therapy can be used to treat people who have endocrine disorders. If you have hypothyroidism, where your thyroid doesn't produce enough hormones, this can be managed by taking a thyroid hormone orally.

People who don't produce enough growth hormone can have developmental problems, but this too can be mitigated with replacement hormones. The same goes for people who have deficiencies in cortisol production, sex hormones, and so on. It isn't just hormones, though, as replacement of albumin, insulin, and clotting factors can all be life-changing or lifesaving therapies.

As great as this is, delivering functional molecules is the least powerful form of replacement. It's relatively safe and convenient thanks to ease of delivery, but we can do more by delivering larger structures.

For example, it's possible to give cells entirely new organelles. This has been done with mitochondria to prevent the transmission of mitochondrial disease from mother to child. During the in vitro fertilization process, mutation-carrying mitochondria in a mother's egg cell can be replaced with healthy mitochondria from a third party. That egg can then be fertilized and the mother will give birth to a child who not only benefits from healthy mitochondria, but—if female—can then pass on healthy mitochondria to her children as well.

Mitochondrial replacement isn't just for embryos, though. Delivering healthy mitochondria to damaged tissues is being tested to help newborns with damaged hearts. Adults might be able to benefit, too. Loss of mitochondrial function occurs with age, and putting healthy mitochondria into an older adult could be beneficial.

The way it works is that young, healthy mitochondria are produced in large batches. These mitochondria are then packaged to facilitate uptake by cells, and injected into the body. Cells that take them up can put them to work, and there have been some early results hinting that this approach could be used to bolster energy-hungry tissues like muscle and the brain.

Mitochondrial replacement is already being commercialized, with many companies developing ways to manufacture and deliver mitochondria. If it turns out to work, this may soon become one of the first true anti-aging interventions that's widely available.

Similar in size to mitochondria are the microbes that live in your digestive tract. These microbes are like a miniature farm that produces helpful nutrients for your body. With age, the good bacteria die off and are replaced with bad bacteria that hurt you instead of helping you. But you can replace the bacteria in your gut with microbiota transplants, also called bacteriotherapy, although the process is currently a little crude.

First, a young, healthy volunteer is found. They are screened and tested for both diseases and healthy levels of gut microbiota. If they pass, then they are asked to collect some of their stool and mail it to people who need it. The recipients then get it into their digestive tract, one way or another. This has been shown to help with certain conditions in humans, like infection with Clostridioides difficile, a bacterium that causes severe diarrhea. It also has been shown to extend lifespan in fish.

However, don't go around making awkward phone calls just yet. Companies are working on developing safer, more controlled alternatives where you can get the bacteria you need, but with much lower risk of getting something you don't want. There will eventually be therapies as powerful as fecal microbiota transplant but as safe as probiotics.

Your human cells can also be replaced, and with more potent effect than the indirect benefits of healthy gut bacteria. Young, healthy cells are great because they can produce healthy enzymes, hormones, and mitochondria. Cell replacement therapy is already available for acute diseases. You can transplant blood stem cells to treat infections and autoimmune diseases. You can also use skin cells to help heal wounds or inject immune cells to help fight cancer and other diseases.

In addition, new cell therapies are being developed that can do even more. Heart muscle cells are being engineered that can go to your heart and help it heal after a heart attack. Brain cell therapies are being developed to treat disorders like Parkinson's disease. Some groups of scientists are working on retinal cells that could restore vision in eye diseases like age-related macular degeneration.

Even these are just the beginning. Once it becomes possible to replenish a cell population periodically, aging damage within that population will be removed and the rejuvenation will have knock-on effects throughout the body. Youthful blood stem cells will produce not just young blood to better support your tissues and organs, but also young immune cells to fight infection and cancer and clear senescent cells more effectively. Young muscle cells will not only protect you from slips and falls, but also improve your metabolism by sending out health-promoting signals called myokines.

Replacing all your cells is much harder than replacing your mitochondria. While mitochondria are essentially the same everywhere in the body, different tissues need specific cell types in specific places. That means cell replacement therapies must produce many different kinds of cells and get each of them to the right location. We know how to do this for some cell types, but not all. If delivery were solved, you could theoretically replace all the cells in your body with younger, healthier versions. You would not even need to replace all 30 trillion cells, because you could instead replace the stem cells that produce your somatic cells, and they would do the rest. That still leaves long-lived cells like neurons and the sensory cells of the inner ear, which will be more difficult to replace—but perhaps still possible, especially if done very gradually.

Cell replacement therapies could help reverse age-related diseases that involve the loss of important cell populations. For example, the age-related loss of muscle mass is partially attributed to the decline in muscle stem cells. Putting in new ones could help you stay strong and metabolically stable. The same goes for a variety of conditions: anemia, immunosenescence, diabetes, and even hair loss. Several neurodegenerative diseases involve the loss of specific cell populations, and replenishing those could help alleviate the conditions.

Many companies are currently attempting replacement with single cell types to treat specific diseases; hopefully over the next few decades this will become a common tool for helping to extend healthy lifespan. However, cell replacement can't be a complete solution because we also need to rejuvenate the extracellular matrix.

What about replacing ECM directly? On a small scale, this is possible. You can grow young, healthy ECM particles in a dish and then inject them into tissue. This young ECM can help cells heal tissue in certain cases, and it has been shown in animals to help repair damage after heart attacks and other injuries. Adding young ECM makes the body younger, but ECM composition varies from tissue to tissue and has precise and intricate structure at the molecular scale. This makes it extremely difficult to inject the right ECM in all the right places. Not to mention that the old ECM would still be present. Even so, it's a good first-generation technology worth some attention and further development. And even if we don't want to immediately start sticking needles in every part of our body, it might be useful to attempt ECM replacement in skin and eventually work our way up to the brain—where it would likely be the most difficult.

ECM replacement can also be done at larger scales. Companies already produce ECM scaffolds that can be implanted to direct tissue healing. The ECM cues cells to rebuild tissue that was lost. This has been shown to work in tissues as different as bone and skin. Common uses for ECM implants today are healing skin wounds, heart muscle patches, bone repair, and giving people new corneas.

Replacing cells and ECM can be combined in a variety of ways. For example, you can seed ECM spheres or scaffolds with young cells. This would help ensure that the cells engraft and, after they do engraft, that they behave like young cells. Cells and ECM are better together. They are best, though, when in their natural configuration, which is hard to recapitulate in the lab.

Of course, you don't have to artificially combine cells and ECM. They naturally occur together in tissues. Anytime you transplant young, healthy tissue you get both healthy cells and healthy ECM. For example, skin grafts are a common treatment for burn victims. They can get skin from donors, or receive skin from unburned parts of their own body. Same-aged skin is better than burned skin, but genetically matched young skin would be even better. Other examples of tissue transplant that are already in use are blood vessel grafts as well as tendons, ligaments, cartilage, and hair.

Body fluids are also replaceable, as we know from blood transfusions. Studies have shown that replacing old blood with young blood can help animals live longer, healthier lives. This is what has been observed in heterochronic parabiosis studies. Heterochronic means different ages, and these studies connected the circulatory systems of young and old animals to see the impact on each animal. What they saw was striking. The younger mouse's body began to perform more like an old body, while the older mouse's body began to perform more like a young one. This rejuvenating effect would probably be true for other fluids as well, including cerebrospinal fluid.

What about replacing organs? If you can swap out an old kidney with a young one, then you will have both young cells and young ECM working for you. The organ will be healthy all the way through, with no disease and no accumulation of aging damage.

Consider the thymus, an organ that trains immune cells. It essentially stops working at the age of 50, and this is part of the reason older people are at greater risk of dying from infection. Transplanting a new thymus would give your adaptive immune system a new lease on life, make vaccines more effective, and potentially increase your healthspan and lifespan. The thymus is one of those organs that can do its job from anywhere in the body, so a new one could be installed in, for example, your abdomen, to make the surgery safer and easier.

Young organs do their jobs more efficiently, are generally less cancer-prone, and also help the rest of the body function better. So if you could swap out lungs, you would not only reduce your chances of chronic obstructive pulmonary disease, but you would be much less likely to develop lung cancer as well.

Plus, each organ replaced would improve the function of the other organs and tissues in your body. A younger heart improves nutrient delivery; a younger liver lowers toxin load and inflammation. So each new organ not only provides direct rejuvenation through new cells and ECM, but also indirect rejuvenation through its effect on the rest of the body.

Organ transplants are already fairly common, with hundreds of thousands of kidneys, tens of thousands of livers, and many hearts, lungs, pancreases, and other organs transplanted each year. These patients have diseases that can't be cured with medicines or other therapies, so surgeons replace the affected organs or tissues with donor material. When the donor is younger than the patient, the patient experiences some level of rejuvenation as well.

Not only can you expand the benefits of replacement by moving toward larger structures like organs, but surgeons have even been moving toward transplanting multiple organs at the same time. Sometimes it's easier to give someone a heart and lungs together rather than one or the other. You also see kidneys transplanted together with the pancreas, and even multivisceral transplants which can include stomach, liver, pancreas, spleen, and small intestine. Today it's also possible to transplant hands, arms, legs, and faces. These large, complex tissue transplants are called vascularized composite allografts.

Modern medicine has a wide array of techniques for replacing molecules, cells, organs, and more. These methods could all potentially be used to treat aging in the near term.

Replacement to Treat Aging

With so many options, where should the limited resources going to replacement be allocated for maximum impact on aging? It is tempting to go all-in on cell therapy, because cells could completely rejuvenate the body. This kind of in situ cellular replacement would be great because cells are relatively easy to produce and relatively easy to get into the body.

For example, if you could get a yearly injection of heart cells that then travel to your heart, take the place of old cells, and replace the local ECM, then you would have a therapy that keeps the heart young and healthy indefinitely. Maybe not all the cells are replaced each year. But what if you can get a 5% replacement rate? Then, on average, your heart will be made of 10-year-old cells and ECM. This sounds pretty good, especially if you started with a heart that had 50 years of damage accumulation.

However, a cell-replacement-based solution to aging faces several technical challenges. First, you need donor cells of many different cell types. Producing different cell types is possible because cells can be coaxed into transforming from one cell type to another, even from somatic cell to stem cell. So, in theory, you could take a few skin cells and produce all the different types of cells you needed for replacement. However, the protocols for doing these cellular transformations aren't yet developed for every cell type, and the existing methods don't always produce perfect results.

The second problem is that you need many cells. Cell expansion is routinely performed in many labs, but some cell types are harder to grow than others. Examples of cells that are hard to multiply in vitro include heart muscle cells, pancreatic beta cells, and liver cells, though there are many others. So even after you have the cell types you want, there's additional work to do to get sufficient quantities of cells for transplantation.

Third, you need a way to get cells to the parts of the body where you want them to go. Some cells will naturally travel to the places in the body where they are supposed to be, but others won't. Hematopoietic stem cells injected intravenously will migrate to bone marrow niches, whereas pancreatic beta cells will simply die in circulation. Cell delivery is therefore another unsolved problem.

Fourth, even if cells reach their target, there's no guarantee they will integrate with the tissue. For example, liver cells might make it to the liver, but then fail to find a spot to take up permanent residence. This is called the engraftment problem, in which cells arrive but don't thrive. This could occur because old cells won't give up their spots, or because old ECM makes the young cells think they are in the wrong place, or simply because some cell types don't have the programming to seek out new places to live.

Fifth, even if you can get some level of engraftment, it isn't guaranteed that you will get uniform replacement of cells within a tissue. For example, if your first dose of replacement cells replaces that 5% of cells that are easiest to reach, the next dose might also be heavily concentrated on the same locations. You could end up replacing the same 5% of an organ over and over, rather than fully rejuvenating it.

Finally, even when all of the preceding challenges are solved, there's still the problem of the extracellular matrix. Some cells do have a limited natural ability to tear down and rebuild ECM around them. It would be convenient if young cells could charge in and rebuild an organ in place. However, cells have not evolved to repair ECM in this way. Even if they were programmed to do so, we know that as ECM accumulates damage, it becomes more difficult for cells to remodel. Chemical cross-links in the ECM, the aggregation of misfolded proteins, or simply wear and tear on long-lived molecules can disrupt cellular function and prevent young cells from doing their jobs well, including maintaining the ECM. That's not to mention that the performance of ECM itself is degraded.

So it may be the case that basic cell therapies will help rejuvenate tissues and organs, but those tissues and organs will eventually fail as the ECM continues to age. Lungs made of young cells, but with old ECM, will still have trouble exhaling. Arteries with young cells, but old ECM, will still be prone to rupture.

Old ECM also has the downside of making young cells less effective. Cells react to their environment, so young cells put onto old ECM start to act like old cells. So while cell replacement therapy can be highly effective for acute diseases, and may have some limited benefits for aging, we will also need some way of replacing the ECM. Cells naturally produce and degrade ECM so, to some extent, cell replacement can also help rejuvenate the ECM. However, there are types of ECM damage that cells aren't equipped to repair. This ECM damage will kill you eventually no matter how young your cells are, so we need alternate solutions.

There's much work to be done to get cell replacement to the point where it can be used to treat aging, and there are also many parallel efforts that could contribute to the eventual success of this approach. Companies are working to harness naturally occurring and modified cells to rejuvenate the body. Many of these therapies currently target specific cell populations for particular diseases, but the technology, techniques, and supporting industry will apply to future therapies as well. There are also specific cell types that naturally try to seek out areas of damage and replace the cells there. We might be able to produce large quantities of these in the lab, and then inject them into patients to clean up certain types of damage throughout their body. Studying them might also give us clues for how to improve cell therapies in general.

However, with no clear path to creating a cell-based solution to aging, we are forced to pursue the more powerful but more dangerous techniques of tissue and organ replacement. To do that, we'll need to solve the two major obstacles to therapeutic replacement: generating the supply of replacement parts and safely delivering them to patients.

Supplying Replacement Parts

Currently, the supply of tissues and organs is very limited, and replacement for longevity would be hard to achieve in today's world of organ shortages. Many companies are working on ways to produce tissues and organs at scale, which would enable a new medical paradigm of replacement. Approaches for the mass production of organs include making them in animals, making them in the lab, and designing artificial organs that can be built in factories.

Animal methods include using regular animal organs, using organs from genetically modified animals, and using human organs grown in animals. Using animal organs in humans is called xenotransplantation. If no human kidney is available, a monkey kidney might be better than nothing. Surprisingly, this actually works to some extent. Unsurprisingly, animal organs tend to lead to immune rejection and have other problems, such as pathogens. That said, the supply of animals is highly scalable, so the approach is being tested and refined. For example, a man was given a pig heart and survived with it for some time.

To make animal organs function better in humans, some groups are genetically modifying them to remove genetic sequences that are dangerous, including genes for proteins that trigger an immune response inside a human body. These changes make this approach work much better than using unmodified animal organs, but not as well as a human organ would.

You can grow a human organ in an animal using a technique called chimerism, where you inject human cells into animal embryos so that some of the animal's organs end up being made of human cells. If you do this in an uncontrolled manner, you end up with organs that are a mix of human and animal cells that is not much better than a regular animal organ. But if you modify the animal cells so that they can't produce a specific organ, then that organ will be made entirely from human cells.

For example, you might use chimerism to produce a pig with human kidneys. Those human kidneys could then be taken out and transplanted into a patient with chronic kidney disease. These organs still tend to have some animal cells and other defects so, while they are better than animal organs, they aren't as good as organs from humans.

In the pursuit of even better organs, laboratory methods are under investigation that include directly building organs with 3D bioprinting and growing organs from cells.

In the case of 3D bioprinting, cells and ECM are dripped in layers to directly build tissues and organs. This approach sometimes works at small scales and for very simple tissues, but struggles with larger and more complex structures. One reason is that while 3D printing allows for the shape of an organ to be mimicked well, it's hard to make small things like blood vessels that the organ needs to function properly.

For some organs, this may be okay because it's unnecessary to fully mimic their natural shape and size in the adult body. Smaller, easier-to-build structures called organoids could potentially be used instead. This would work especially well for organs that don't need to be in a specific location to do their job. For example, instead of having a single thymus the size of a walnut, you might install a dozen pea-sized thymus organoids that could mature T cells at the same overall rate.

Another problem with 3D bioprinting is that it's a bit like putting a tree back on its stump after being cut down. It may look similar, but the molecular connections to hold it together aren't all there. Cells can rebuild the connections to some extent, but not as well as when a tree or organ grows naturally.

Growing organs from cells, on the other hand, taps the development programs in our DNA to create perfect replacement organs. Tissue or organs can be grown to size in a bioreactor, which is just a high-tech jar of fluid for growing cells. Growing human organs in bioreactors would be very scalable, but it's hard to get cells to grow into an organ outside of the context of a developing human body. The organs of your body are meant to work together as a team. If you try to grow a kidney by itself, your bioreactor has to supply the oxygen that would normally come from the lungs, the blood flow that would normally come from the heart, and so on. Bioreactors can do this to some extent, but they can't beat the real thing.

Fortunately, they don't have to. A new approach has been developed that flips organ interdependence from a problem to a solution. Specifically, if you grow a set of organs together, then they can support each other just as they evolved to, which minimizes the amount of work the bioreactor needs to do. This means that growing multiple organs at once can actually be much easier than growing just one.

To do this, you take a cell or a group of cells and instruct them to follow the same developmental process that produces a full organism. Every cell has this program in its DNA, and it can be activated by stimulating the right genes. Before getting started, though, you genetically edit the cells so they will produce only the tissues and organs you want.

There are two ways to coax adult cells into following the developmental program. The first is somatic cell nuclear transfer, where you combine the nucleus of an adult cell with an egg cell that has had its nucleus removed. Molecular cues in the egg cell reset the adult nucleus, allowing it to start the developmental process.

You don't have to use egg cells, though. Scientists have identified the molecular cues in egg cells and can use just those to get adult cells like skin cells to do the same thing. The second method uses those cues to instruct adult cells to form what's called an "embryoid" model.

These embryoids are being investigated for making cell types that could be useful for cell therapies, such as treating Parkinson's disease. However, if they are grown longer, they might eventually be used to make organs as well. So you effectively say, "Hey, grow like you normally would, but only produce a heart, lungs, kidneys, etc."

The trick here is that you should not tell them to build only a kidney, because a kidney can't survive on its own. For this approach to work, you need to give genetic instructions that allow a set of organs to grow together. It isn't currently known what the minimum set of organs is that can be successfully produced in this way. But, given the current organ shortage, the more the merrier.

If you built only the internal organs of the torso, the result might be called a visceral organ construct. Visceral organ constructs might be used like organ donors today, where individual organs are shared among many patients. One visceral organ construct could help a dozen people. Or they could be used for multi-organ transplants for one or two patients. Either way, they would radically change both the supply of organs and the way we think about treating disease.

Multi-organ constructs would also help accelerate medical progress by providing testing platforms for new therapies. If you have a drug that improves heart health, and you test it on people, you could potentially have acute side effects or even kill someone. Instead, you can test the drug in organ constructs to see how the organs respond before you give it to a person. This would not only make drugs and other medical interventions safer, but make research and development much faster and cheaper. Doctors would get access to more new medicines each year, as well as higher confidence that the medicines would help their patients.

Growing organs may make people feel uncomfortable, just as heart transplants originally did. Unfortunately, we do not have a choice between growing organs or not. We have a choice between growing them or accepting a death sentence for every person who could otherwise be saved. Keep in mind that the first organs grown will be small, so the first patients who will either be saved or left to die will be young children.

Bodyoids

There's no reason to limit ourselves to internal organs. Suppose a firefighter lost their foot saving a family from a burning building. It would be wonderful if we could grow a new foot that could then be transplanted. However, you wouldn't be growing a foot in isolation. What you would do is grow internal organs and a leg together. You could then take the foot for the firefighter and donate the other parts to people who need them.

Using this hypothetical technology, the maximum amount of tissue that can be grown without creating a new person is called a bodyoid.

While a bodyoid would not have a brain that could produce a person, it would have internal organs, legs, arms, and a head. You might grow some sub-structures of the brain, say the ones necessary for regulating automatic breathing or secreting certain hormones. However, you would not include the parts of the brain needed to develop thinking or feeling.

Bodyoids are the most complete solution to supply because you could get just about anything you might need to help someone who is sick or injured. These constructs would give a wide range of options for rejuvenating the body. A new pair of legs could increase mobility and bring related benefits from increased exercise, socializing, self-care, and metabolism. New arms could be the difference between independence and living in a care center.

In a world where young, immune-matched bodyoids are available, medicine would look very different. There would be no organ shortage, no waiting lists, nobody hoping that someone else will die so that they don't have to. There would also be enough blood for every emergency room and operating room because each bodyoid could donate regularly to blood banks. In addition, bodyoids could be used for parabiosis. The more competent immune system and regulatory systems of the bodyoid could help improve a patient's health ahead of organ transplants to improve outcomes, or at any time a patient needs a health boost. Simply having access to a young thymus via shared circulation could lead to real benefits in patient health.

Bodyoids could also provide donor tissue for spinal cord repair and help treat the millions of people living with chronic spinal cord injury. Skin grafts would be available to treat burns. And for those in dangerous professions, new hands, arms, and legs would be available when necessary.

Another benefit of bodyoids is truly personalized medicine. When you have a set of human organs you can test therapies on, you can make much more rapid progress. You could actually see the impact of a treatment before applying it to yourself. This wouldn't be perfect given the age difference and lack of most brain tissues, but you would have a much better sense than you would get from testing in animals. Biotech companies could move much faster by running clinical trials on tissue constructs rather than real people. You might not even need clinical trials if you could directly test an intervention on bodyoids before giving it to patients.

The most comprehensive replacement approach requires large-scale tissue replacement, so a major focus for radical life extension should be on the production of the largest, most complex human tissue constructs we can manage. This may mean multi-organ constructs that would allow us to replace most of the internal organs, or it might consist of bodyoids that would provide almost every organ and tissue in the body. Replacing one's entire old body with a young one is the most impactful single aging intervention that has been plausibly conceived of.

While we want to produce as much replacement material as possible, there's an ethical line that can't be crossed. If you accidentally produced a bodyoid with a functioning brain, it could become a person, and would no longer be an ethical source for donor materials. So as human tissue constructs are used to develop more of the body, it's important to ensure that their development can only go so far. Specifically, you need to ensure that the construct can't produce the parts of the brain that might contribute to the creation of a mind—a thinking, feeling individual who would own the tissues and be harmed by losing parts of their body.

Something similar happens naturally in a small percentage of human pregnancies due to random genetic defects. In cases of anencephaly, a body develops from an embryo without a full brain. When there is no brain, there's no chance for a person to develop, but the organs can still be healthy. There have been a few rare cases of anencephaly where parents opted to have the organs donated to save the lives of babies who needed them. The natural examples of anencephaly are highly variable in what parts of the brain do form, so simply replicating them isn't sufficient for ethical bodyoid production. What must be strived for is highly robust and failsafe methods for exactly making only the tissues you want, and nothing else.

Preventing cells from producing neural tissue relies on genetic editing techniques that already exist. In the simplest case, certain genes necessary for brain tissue are either removed from cells before they are used to grow a body or DNA is added that encodes a self-destruct signal. In the first case, you're making it so that cells can't go down developmental pathways to produce a brain. In the latter case, you're ensuring that any cells that decide to turn into brain cells go through programmed cell death, called apoptosis. All of these techniques are aimed at ensuring that no mind develops.

It's also important to ensure that the genetic changes that produce brainless bodyoids are robust. You would not want to depend on a single genetic edit because biology is messy and unpredictable. It would be much better to have several methods that work independently, so that even if one fails, you won't end up with a body inhabited by a person.

There are many genes that can prevent parts or all of the brain from growing. Current research is looking into what options are available in different species. What works in animals won't always directly translate to humans, but the technology has immediate applications. You could, for example, reduce suffering by creating brainless livestock or brainless animals for testing drugs and other interventions. It may seem strange to create an animal bodyoid for experimentation, but it's clearly better than using animals that can experience pain.

Bodyoid technology is still in its early stages, but there have been encouraging results. Visceral organ constructs have been produced with mouse cells. Separately, it was shown that it's possible to disable genetic pathways that lead to the development of a head, and this can be done in a way that ensures no brain is produced.

Support Systems

Once you have a construct ready, you need a place for it to grow. While an organoid can be grown in a small container and absorb oxygen and nutrients through diffusion, a large bodyoid would need a sophisticated support system. The most reliable approach is to have it form something like a placenta and then attach that placenta to an ectogenesis system.

Ectogenesis technology mimics what happens inside a mammalian womb. It's a special kind of bioreactor that creates a healthy environment for growth. Think of a large glass cylinder filled with fluid. There would be a large gel pad on the side, which the placenta could grow on and into. This pad would have three key properties. First, it would be large enough to accommodate the placenta's maximum size at full maturity.

Second, it would be made of special materials that allow the placenta to grow into it, just like the side of a uterus. Third, it would have artificial vasculature circulating oxygen- and nutrient-rich fluids that allow for the exchange of molecules and gases with the construct's circulatory system.

Prototypes of artificial wombs have been shown to work in the early stages of human embryo development as well as during the first few weeks for other animals. They are also effective in the later stages of development when animals are approaching birth. However, there's still a technological gap for the intermediate period; nobody has yet succeeded in growing a mammal in such an artificial system from a single cell to birth.

A fully fledged system would support the growth of the bodyoid as it runs through the developmental program and creates new types of cells and tissues along the way. However, this is no easy task, because the final product is roughly a billion times larger than the starting cells. That's like going from an origami boat to an oil tanker.

The bioreactor would also need to dynamically adjust the nutrients and molecular signals to match what organs are normally exposed to as they grow. This means it needs special monitoring systems and the ability to change the contents of both the fluid surrounding the construct and the reagent that exchanges molecules and gases with the placenta.

On top of that, the system needs to be kept sterile for many months. This is beyond a typical upper limit of what is currently achieved, but specialized systems should be able to push that limit out to what is needed. While not currently ready, ectogenesis technology is close enough that a determined push could bring it to maturity relatively quickly.

Artificial wombs can only take development so far, producing small-sized constructs with small-sized organs. That's okay, because small parts are perfect for helping babies and young children. So even if adults might need to wait, we don't need to wait to start saving lives. Even adults can benefit from small organs, which usually have extra capacity. Some organs, like livers and kidneys, can even finish growing in size after they are transplanted.

Producing large bodyoids would require additional support to reach adult size in good condition. Things that would need to be figured out include monitoring, food and waste management, and keeping the constructs healthy. This might be done in specialized chambers, perhaps similar to the equipment used today to care for people in comas. We already have technology that can monitor vital signs in real time. To keep those biomarkers strong, bodyoids would need exercise. Electrical stimulation of the muscles might keep them from atrophying, but it would be better to use the bodyoid nervous system. This would help maintain the nerve connections and actually lead to stronger muscles. Perhaps a neural-computer interface that attaches to the upper spinal cord could do this by taking the place of the missing brain. Exercise would also help maintain strong bones, a healthy cardiovascular system, etc.

There's some concern that a person might die while waiting for replacement organs to be big enough. This is a real concern, but not for the reasons you might expect. Small organs generally have the capacity to support much larger bodies than they typically reside in. For example, the kidneys of a five-year-old could support the body of an adult. So, if the need arose, someone might opt to use tissue or organs that weren't yet fully developed. Furthermore, once the industry is scaled, parts of all sizes will be available on demand, so the sooner we get started the better.

While an undersized pancreas might be just fine, there are organs that would be better to wait on. For example, spinal cords have an organized cross-sectional structure. If you wanted to replace a length of spinal cord, it would be much easier to successfully transplant it if the cross-sections were close in size. Hearts also need to be big enough to support a patient's body.

If you have time and money, the first donor bodyoids produced will probably be made to order for early adopters. The exact genetic match will ensure correct sizing of any parts as well as immune compatibility. In the long run, though, it will be preferable to have a set of mass-produced, inexpensive bodyoids that can be matched to a patient, treated for immune compatibility, and used immediately, rather than waiting for genetically identical donor material.

Modulating the immune response is a common part of transplant procedures today, and there are techniques for making it easier for patients to live with donor tissues and organs. One of the newest methods involves giving the patient some of the donor's bone marrow in addition to whatever else is transplanted. This bone marrow then produces immune cells that help protect the transplanted tissues from the patient's immune system. It may seem a little strange to have two immune systems, but as long as they can get along, it's a much better situation than being dependent on immune-suppressing drugs. This approach has already been successfully used in humans to achieve full immunocompatibility of transplants without immunosuppression, and will likely become standard as the techniques involved mature.

Another concern is that human bodyoids might not scale quickly enough to have an impact. The total demand for bodyoids alone might be in the hundreds of millions per year. It's a daunting task. But it isn't all or nothing. Constructs intended for creating different cell types are relatively small and fast to grow, so they could start treating diseases quickly and scale to reach millions of people in a few years. Visceral organ constructs and bodyoids are slower and more capital-intensive. However, even if it takes five years to get to production rates in the tens of thousands, you will still have solved the organ shortage for children and newborns. That alone makes it worthwhile. If it takes another 10 years to reach all the adults, that would still be a huge success.

Bodyoids require the most time and effort to grow, but their care can be provided periodically and without much human intervention. The periods of greatest activity would be when their initial cells are created and modified, when the resulting cells are placed in an artificial womb, and finally when the bodyoid is placed into a maturation device.

It would be convenient if bodyoids could serve as incubators for more bodyoids. Unfortunately, new bodyoids would take many years to reach the size to act as incubators; while you're waiting, you aren't getting much improvement in supply. It might be faster and more economical to mature artificial womb technology in that time period. Another alternative is to develop techniques for growing bodyoids inside animals. For example, if you develop a construct that has human cells for most of the tissue and organs, but animal cells for the placenta, then animals could be used to grow replacement parts for humans in a more conscientious way than recovering human organs from chimeric animals.

There's also the possibility of genetically engineering the constructs to mature faster, potentially saving time and money. Examples of accelerated growth are seen in conditions like Sotos syndrome, Weaver syndrome, and gigantism. However, this would need to be tested for its long-term impact on the quality of tissues and organs.

Artificial Replacement

Replacement has one more tactic to solve the supply problem, and that's artificial replacement parts. There's a long history of replacing biological functions with artificial substitutes. Hips, teeth, and hearts are just some of the body parts for which artificial versions are available. Artificial replacement has the benefit of unlimited supply because components can be manufactured to meet any demand. Some artificial replacements can perform just as well as their biological counterparts and, because they are made with technology that's fully understood, continue to improve rapidly over time.

For example, it's currently possible to replace the lens in your eye with an implantable intraocular lens. This can treat and prevent cataracts, but there are new lenses in testing that would allow recipients to see about three times better than 20/20 vision. Similarly, emerging hearing aids with noise cancellation and directional focus can help people hear more clearly than those with normal hearing. Artificial hearts may eventually be preferable to their biological counterparts, as they will be immune to fatigue, ischemia, infection, and aging.

However, most artificial replacements are currently not as good as their biological counterparts. An artificial leg might help you walk, but it won't be quite as dexterous or provide the same sensory feedback. It also doesn't give you the benefit of myokine signaling and metabolic effects from leg muscles or a supply of blood and immune cells from bone marrow. In many cases, artificial replacement isn't yet even an option. A dialysis machine can replace some of the blood filtering capabilities of a kidney, but not its endocrine functions. Similarly, insulin pumps can help replace some of the endocrine functions of the pancreas, but they don't help with exocrine functions like the production of digestive enzymes. And we have only partial or temporary replacements for lungs, liver, and other organs.

It would be extremely useful to be able to supply all the life support functions of the body through machines. True artificial organs would end the organ shortage, but you don't need organ-sized machines to obtain most of the benefit. Even if you had a dialysis-sized machine for each organ, you would be able to restore any essential function in a hospital setting. For the purposes of radical life extension, this could be just as effective as transplanting young organs, though without the surgical risk. You'd be stuck in the hospital, but there are worse places to be trapped if you're trying to live as long as possible.

In theory, artificial replacement of the brain could be achievable, but this currently seems so distant that it can't factor into the plans of those living today. Still, it makes sense to pursue artificial replacement opportunistically wherever it has a relative advantage. If parts of the brain are amenable to generic replacement, why not consider giving someone an artificial cerebellum?

Overall, for the foreseeable future, replacement will be primarily based on biological materials, and producing those biological materials is the biggest bottleneck to therapeutic replacement.

Delivering Replacement Parts

Once the supply of tissues and organs is secured, it's clear how to use them. Take care of everyone on the waiting lists, and expand usage to anyone who could benefit from, for example, a new pair of kidneys. Then start using organs more proactively, and in larger combinations.

As the supply side begins to catch up with demand, the delivery side of the equation will become more important. If young organs are available, why wait for a heart attack when you can put in a young heart? The answer is that any surgery carries risks of complications and death, and you have to weigh the costs and benefits of any therapy before trying it.

Transplants come with risks far greater than cell therapy, especially when they involve internal organs. In current clinical practice, the mortality rates can be quite high, with procedures like lung transplants reaching as high as 25%. While most of the risk is due to underlying conditions rather than the surgery itself, age is a risk factor and complications like bleeding and infection carry a significant risk of death for any major surgery. So if a single surgery is dangerous and potentially life-threatening, getting repeated surgeries to replace your kidneys, heart, lungs, liver, and so on would be even more dangerous. Of course, not replacing your organs is also dangerous, because you will eventually age to death, but is there a safer way to get new tissues and organs? How can we maximize the benefits of replacement while minimizing the dangers?

One way to minimize surgical risk is to develop autonomous robotic surgical platforms. Robotics and AI have achieved superhuman performance in many areas, and they could do the same for transplant surgeries. Unmatched speed, dexterity, perception, and knowledge have already been demonstrated in many forms of physical automation, and while surgery has unique challenges, it seems likely that transplant surgeons who use this emerging technology will be able to achieve higher survival rates and better outcomes, and make replacement procedures a viable option for more and more people.

Another strategy for reducing surgical risk is to perform fewer surgeries. This can be done by simply transplanting more tissue in a single operation. Surgeons already prefer to transplant combinations of organs in some cases, like transplanting a heart along with lungs. If your goal is to get a new set of internal organs, it might be safer and easier to transplant all of them in a single operation rather than undergoing a dozen individual operations. That way, you only need to worry about the major inputs and outputs to the organ network. Just think of all the connections between organs that can be kept healthy and intact when they are transplanted together.

But there's another consideration, which is that, just as young cells put into old ECM don't function well, young organs put into an old body don't function as well as they would in a young body. This is because of the signaling that happens between different organs. The bloodstream of an old body is full of confusing signals and inflammation that disrupt organ function.

When your car's brakes start to wear out, you replace them before it gets too dangerous to drive. Similarly, you would probably want to replace your heart before the risk of heart failure gets too high. Unfortunately, while new brakes work perfectly, young organs put into an old body won't work as well as they would in a young one.

Fortunately, with enough replacement you can tip things the other way. Give an older person enough young tissues and organs and you can flip the balance of the system, letting youthful signals dominate and rejuvenate the remaining older tissue. The key question is how much replacement is needed to cross that threshold—the therapeutic window for aging replacement.

Replacing only your toes would not meaningfully change your lifespan, but having a young pair of legs might have some impact. Certainly getting a young set of internal organs could add many years to your life. To get the maximum benefit, you would want to replace as much of your body as possible.

This multi-organ transplant strategy meshes nicely with producing organs as integrated organ networks rather than individually. If it's easier to grow organs together, and safer to transplant them together, then there's a natural efficiency to the process. You would produce as many organs as you can in a single batch, perhaps all of the internal organs, and then give them to a recipient at the same time. This might seem aggressive, but patients have already received up to eight organs in a single operation, so it isn't outlandish to think that all the internal organs could be transplanted at once.

This idea of getting as much young tissue as possible for the lowest possible surgical risk can be taken to the extreme with a brain transplant. In this hypothetical procedure, a full bodyoid is produced, and then the patient's brain is removed from their old, damaged body and placed into the young, healthy body. The brain would then enjoy the benefits of young kidneys, a young liver, a young immune system, and so on.

The idea isn't entirely far-fetched, as scientists have been able to keep animal brains biologically active outside of their original bodies for days by perfusing them with oxygenated blood. However, it's much easier to remove a brain from a body than to put one back in again. Implanting a brain would involve numerous challenging vascular and nerve reconnections that would have to happen inside the skull or in another vulnerable position. With sufficiently advanced robotics technology it could be done, but currently the surgical risk would be so high that it would outweigh the benefits.

Body Transplants

In the near term, to maximize benefits while minimizing surgical risk, the likely optimal balance would be to operate at the level of the neck. In this case, instead of keeping just their brain, a patient would keep their entire head and be given a new body from the neck down. Doing a body transplant at the neck has the advantage that all of the connections are stretched along the neck into long lengths that are easier to work with and are mainly covered by soft tissue. This makes the surgery faster and easier, which would translate to relatively high survival rates. Functional outcomes should also be improved since the nerves can more easily be accessed for reconnection. It would still be dangerous, but desperate times call for desperate measures.

A body recipient would enjoy not only a young, healthy set of internal organs, but also young skin, skeletal muscle, and bones. After a period of recovery and rehabilitation, the person would be biologically much younger and healthier, enjoying full rejuvenation from the neck down.

Some people may wonder if they will look strange with an old head and a young body. Yes, but bodyoids would produce the tissue necessary to replace skin above the neck as well, which would not only look nicer but also provide better protection against injuries, infection, cancer, and so on. You'd probably want not just young skin, but every tissue that can be transplanted. Young eyes will see better. A young jaw will have less tooth wear and decay. Maybe parts of the skull could be replaced at the same time to facilitate access to the brain for longevity treatments. These above-the-neck procedures would probably follow a recovery period from the main surgery, but a more chronologically cohesive appearance would be worth the wait.

Body transplants would preserve a patient's brain so that there's no impact on their memories or personality, while giving the patient full rejuvenation of every other aspect of their biology. They would get a new heart, lungs, immune system, etc., while eliminating the baggage of an old body: inflammation, cancer, metabolic problems, and so on.

In addition, the patient's brain would likely benefit. Having the support of a young body might make it so that the brain could continue to function in good health for longer than when attached to an aging body. While it would not solve all the problems of an aging brain, it could help partially reverse or delay the onset of age-related conditions like neurodegeneration.

While difficult, risky, and expensive at first, this would simultaneously solve some of the most challenging diseases. It would also be the only option available for many people with the most serious conditions who have no other treatment options. Multi-organ failure, metastatic cancer, and many other terrible diseases could all be resolved in the same way. Accidental injuries that would otherwise be fatal could become fully recoverable. If a surgeon said they could give you a younger, healthier body with a 50% chance of survival, would you take the risk? Perhaps not, but someone with a terminal condition might. And it just so happens that all of us have a terminal condition called aging.

Beyond curing diseases and reversing aging, body transplant technology would offer two additional benefits. First, if you grow a bodyoid from scratch, then you can perform genetic edits to the original cells used to grow it, and those changes will be present throughout the donor bodyoid. It is much harder to deliver genetic edits throughout a patient's existing body, so replacement may become the fastest way to provide advanced bioengineering therapies.

The second is that body transplants will likely be part of the solution for reviving those who enter biostasis. If you put life on pause with cryonics, you likely have either a body that's aged and diseased or no body at all if you chose head or brain-only preservation. Naturally, a new body would solve both of those problems. The cells to create the bodyoid could be extracted while you are in stasis.

Bodyoids aren't the only solution for revival, as artificial organs could be used to bring you back online. But, even if you theoretically could be a head in a jar, being revived in a human body will probably have some psychological benefits. You'll be dealing with enough as it is with skipping a long period of history and waking up suddenly in a new time, with new technology and new culture.

That's all great, but actually getting body transplants to work has two key requirements. First, the patient must survive decapitation, which is normally lethal. Second, they must recover motor and autonomic function after a complete spinal cord injury, which is widely considered impossible.

Transplanting an entire body may seem like science fiction, but the concept has already been tested in animals. In the 20th century, surgeons showed that a dog's head could survive after being grafted onto another dog's body. Another surgical team showed that a monkey could survive after having its body removed and replaced with another monkey's body.

More recently, survival after body transplantation was shown to work in mice as well. In all of these cases, however, instead of reconnecting all the neck tissues as would be required in a complete body transplant, only certain tissues were reconnected. This means that circulation between the head and donor body was working, but the nerves weren't reconnected. The tests were also limited by the amount of support the animals received compared to what would be given to a human patient, such as immunosuppressants. Despite these limitations, the animals survived the surgery, and some lived for days or weeks afterward.

Survival is important, but it's also important to show that the patient will be able to use the body after the procedure. To do this, recent work has focused on functional recovery. Studies on rodents, dogs, sheep, and pigs have shown that severed spinal cords can be fused back together and that paralyzed animals can learn to walk again.

Normally spinal cords can't be repaired, because damage from car accidents or other blunt force trauma causes cell death and scarring along the length of the spinal cord. This prevents the nerve cells in your spine from healing. However, if you carefully transect a spinal cord with a sharp blade and immediately apply medication, the two ends can fuse back together and begin working again. Thus, in the case of surgically transected spinal cords in a controlled setting, the damage is highly localized and uniform. This makes it relatively easy to repair, which is exactly what you need in a body transplant.

Immediately after the surgery, a patient will be completely paralyzed and dependent on external life support. However, recent spinal fusion research suggests that after a recovery period they will be able to walk, eat, and generally live a normal life. In mice, it takes about a week to start walking again. Rats take two weeks. Larger animals, like pigs, need eight weeks. However, that's with current technology. There are new medications in development that appear to speed up the healing process.

Despite this promising data, there's a long way to go before body transplants can be used to help people in clinical practice. There are cranial and spinal nerves that need to be fused as well, such as the vagus nerves, phrenic nerves, and sympathetic trunks. You will also want to make sure muscles cut during surgery reconnect properly so your extended lifespan isn't accompanied by an annoying stiff neck.

In practice, this means we need a lot more experience doing the kinds of neck surgery that would be needed. New tools and techniques need to be developed for rapid tissue welding and life support during the long surgery. These need to be tested in realistic scenarios, ideally with animal bodyoids, in which older animals will be given young bodies and then tracked to see the impact on biomarkers, healthspan, and lifespan. If things go well, we could try the process on older animals to study the rejuvenating effect on the brains of the recipients. All of this will inform when full-body transplants are ready to attempt as a therapy for humans.

Machines that can support life while the body is nonfunctional will also improve outcomes. Better extracorporeal membrane oxygenation machines would enable tissues to get the oxygen they need to survive while circulation is disconnected and reconnected between the patient's body and the donor body. In fact, technology to keep isolated brain tissue alive and metabolically active for many hours without a body has already been demonstrated, and is continuing to advance.

Body transplants aren't a magic bullet for aging. Current transplant surgeries are dangerous and take their toll on patients. Body transplants will be even more challenging. After a body transplant, you would face a long recovery: weeks in bed while your neck heals, then months or years of physical therapy to master your new body and its unfamiliar neural connections, with help along the way for pain, wound care, and emotional support. But you would go through all of it with the benefit of a young body, a young immune system, and, hopefully, a renewed sense of optimism.

Scaling Replacement

As new supplies of organs are created, human surgeons will be able to absorb the initial increase in organ and tissue availability, but they will not be able to meet demand in a world where organs are no longer scarce. Training enough surgeons isn't feasible, and even if we had 10 times the number of transplant surgeons, it would not be enough personnel to help everyone. Another problem is that a body transplant surgery is extremely complex and time-sensitive. When a mock body transplant procedure was performed by a surgical team, it took 18 hours to complete. It would be challenging even to retrain the existing surgeons on this new procedure.

The only way to reach everyone is to automate transplantation with robotics. As with laser eye surgery, you could have a machine that does most of the work and is supervised by human staff. Machines can be duplicated much more quickly than human doctors, so instead of having a team of surgeons perform each surgery, it would be better for each surgeon to run a surgery by themselves using a machine, or perhaps supervise a team of technicians who are each running machines and only step in when there's a complication.

In this scenario, you would need only about 10,000 machines operating 24/7 to satisfy worldwide demand. If this seems like a large number of machines, consider that more than twice as many commercial aircraft are currently in service around the world. Body transplant robots might also be similar in cost to airplanes, so the airline industry might be a good point of reference for the cost and complexity of creating a body transplant industry.

However, no matter how well body transplants work and how young and healthy your body is, there is still the problem of brain aging.

Brain Replacement

The impact that a body transplant would have on lifespan is still unknown. With most heart disease, cancer, and metabolic diseases resolved, people might expect to live many additional years. Those might be good years indeed, with the wisdom of advanced age combined with the strength and energy of youth. Hopefully there will soon be studies on heterochronic body transplantation in animals to see the effect of giving an old animal a young body on biomarkers, healthspan, and lifespan.

However, even if you replace everything but the brain, that isn't a complete solution. A young body on its own might last an additional 50 years, but a brain that continues to age will greatly limit how much additional time you would survive.

With the brain as the limiting factor, a pessimistic view would be that brain aging would kill you at roughly the same age as before. An optimistic view would be that, because the body is the brain's support system, having young kidneys, a young liver, and a young immune system might add many years to the life of your brain, and thus your life as well.

Still, eventually the vasculature in your brain will break, and you will die from aneurysms and strokes—or from brain cancer or some neurodegenerative disease. Maybe all of this happens 20 years later than it normally would. Twenty years is wonderful, but for the goal of radical life extension, it can only ever be part of the plan. Eventually the brain would need to be rejuvenated as well.

The brain is an especially hard case, because its structure contains the person we're trying to save. The brain is where you live, so it can't be replaced wholesale without killing the patient. There is no clear-cut solution but, despite this, there are still two strategies for replacing the brain.

First, it would be most convenient if cell-based replacement could work. If you could slowly add young neurons and supporting cells that can integrate and take over for the old cells, that might help extend the healthspan and lifespan of the brain. You lose tens of thousands of brain cells every day, so don't be too alarmed at the prospect of new cells moving in and taking over. The human brain shrinks considerably as you age; it's about 10-20% smaller in your 70s and 80s. If used properly, new cells could help boost your brain and make it easier to remember where you left your glasses.

The major challenge with this cellular replacement of the brain, as with all tissues, is the problem of repairing the extracellular matrix. In some sense the brain's ECM might be easier for cells to replace because it contains much less elastin, and also experiences much less mechanical stress, compared to organs like the lungs. On the other hand, the brain's ECM supports delicate structures that help define memories and other brain functions, so more care is needed when trying to replace it. It's perhaps possible to transplant not just cells but also small volumes of young ECM, but it isn't yet clear if or how that would work.

In the cell-based replacement scenario, you would receive a yearly injection of cells that would travel to your brain and integrate into the existing network. The specific cells you use to see, hear, or remember your name might change over time, but you would retain all the same functions and memories. With luck, some of the cells would help rebuild at least portions of the ECM of the brain to make sure the new cells have a healthy environment in which to live and work.

Due to the centrality of the brain, all avenues to its rejuvenation should be pursued. If, as current evidence suggests, it turns out that cells can't fix the ECM, integrate, or take over for old cells, then more drastic approaches might be needed.

One proposal is progressive brain replacement with tissue transplants, a concept developed by Jean Hébert and described in his book *Replacing Aging*. In this scenario, discrete volumes of brain matter would be slowly silenced, then taken out and replaced with young tissue that can integrate with the host brain. You might, for example, replace one of the wrinkles of your neocortex with a small disk of precursor tissue. That tissue can grow into a new mound of cortical tissue, sort of like those compressed towels that expand when you get them wet. If you did this slowly over time, perhaps 5% of the brain per year, then every 20 years you would have a fully replaced brain. Because the brain shrinks with age, the amount of tissue to be silenced and removed would be less than what is being added.

The new tissue would require time to take over important functions of the brain, and there would need to be an equally slow loss of function from any tissue before removal. For example, you might gently turn off the region that's responsible for hearing over the course of a year. You would not notice this, because the hearing functions would be moved automatically to other parts of the brain. Once the target region was no longer doing any work, it would be taken out and replaced with young tissue. That young tissue would then fill the gap and begin to take over some of the brain's workload.

Neuroplasticity, the ability of the brain to change where certain processing happens, is the reason that progressive brain replacement could work while replacing all of the brain at once would not. Going piece by piece allows the brain time to adapt and move functions, at least in theory.

There's a good basis for this theory, though. People who develop tumors in their brain often lose regions associated with speech or other functions that they use in their day to day lives. However, if the tumor grows slowly, then they may never notice any problems. Their speech is sometimes maintained at the same level as it's moved to other parts of the brain during tumor growth. This happens in real cases and shows the enormous power of brain plasticity.

The slow, progressive replacement is needed for areas of the brain that contribute to individuality rather than just handling basic functions. The former can't be regrown without changing who you are: hippocampus, amygdala, prefrontal cortex, temporal lobes, and limbic system. On the other hand, there are potential opportunities to more aggressively replace more generic parts of the brain: medulla oblongata, pons, primary motor cortex, and primary visual cortex. They are all important, but if you had an off-the-shelf version you could potentially swap those in without changing who you are.

Even more aggressive proposals have been considered as well. Much of the brain is divided into semi-separate halves that behave somewhat redundantly. For example, you might be able to take out half of your cerebellum at a time. Applying this approach to various structures could potentially speed up the replacement of the brain, and make the process safer and more effective.

Of course, even if you can grow young tissue grafts to put in, the process of transplantation in the brain is a dangerous and complicated proposition. There are four major hurdles.

The first is removing the tissue you want to replace. Instead of simply adding cells, reinforcing neural circuits, and repopulating cell groups, tissue transplants require the bulk removal of cells. The surgery for this is somewhat complicated because you don't want to cause bleeding or damage any surrounding regions. If that weren't hard enough, you have to disable the regions you want to remove before you do so. If you don't properly silence the regions you want to remove, then you can cause major damage. Any time you remove tissue volumes, you run the risk of damaging structures that contain important parts of who you are. What is worse is that the highly interconnected nature of the brain makes it difficult to limit the damage. Neural projections from many parts of the brain might run through the same small volume of tissue, so destroying it could impact many different brain functions. So safe methods of turning off a volume of brain before removing it would be crucial.

The second hurdle is getting the replacement tissue in. Surgically you can try to stick a piece of tissue in place, but without proper blood supply it will die. Even if you can get it in place and supported, the highly interconnected nature of the brain makes it difficult to simply replace one region and restore the original function. The new tissue would need to reach out to all the other parts of the brain that it was previously connected to, as well as to draw in connections from various places.

However, if you regrow a volume of tissue using the normal developmental process, new vasculature can be created as needed and immature neurons will connect extensively with the rest of the brain. Whether all the necessary connections form in this context is unknown, as normally the brain all grows together—so more research may be necessary to find ways of getting those connections to form.

Third, this approach requires routine brain surgery. Having your body cut off and replaced is risky and invasive, but you would probably only have to do it once. Opening up the skull and operating inside it carries serious risk, and undergoing that risk every few years creates low odds of long-term survival. Even with a cryonics contract in place, you should try to avoid risky situations.

Finally, while the above is a plausible strategy for the neocortex, it isn't clear that it will work for other brain regions. Can you progressively replace your midbrain? Is it even feasible to access it for surgical replacement? It isn't clear that every region of the brain is as plastic as the sensory and motor cortex. Can memories and personalities move as easily? Some interesting experiments will be needed to find out.

There are many things to try, and the more we push the limits of tissue replacement for the brain, the more we will learn about opportunities and limitations for different approaches. For example, could you gradually silence an entire half of the brain and replace one hemisphere at a time? More work is needed to find out how far this approach can go.

Unfortunately, the immediate prospects for brain replacement aren't so good. However, even partial solutions could be highly impactful. If we can get brain replacement to work completely, then in combination with body transplantation, we will have a full solution to the problem of aging.

Key Takeaways

When considering how best to allocate your time and effort for radical life extension, replacement should be high on your list. Not only could it be a complete solution to aging, but it currently appears to be both the nearest and least expensive solution. So any time and money devoted to replacement would be well spent, as it would go into the most efficient strategy for saving lives.

This is because replacement sidesteps the difficulties associated with solving aging with drugs, which are limited by our understanding of biology. Replacement is an inherently complete solution to aging damage for the part being replaced, eliminates both diseases and aging, and scales to the whole body and maybe even the brain. The strategy of growing young, healthy cells, tissues, and organs and then transplanting them into patients is a shortcut around the decades or more of work required to comprehensively understand and engineer solutions to aging processes. Replacement also benefits from the option of using synthetic substitutes, which often have special advantages of their own.

The advantages of replacement can already be seen in modern transplant practice: when doctors can't cure liver disease, they give patients a new liver. So we know it's often easier to replace organs than to cure the underlying disease. If this is true for a single illness in a single organ, imagine how much more the balance shifts for aging, which is a process orders of magnitude more complex and spans every tissue and organ in the body.

Some types of replacement have the downside of requiring surgery. For radical life extension, you want to get as much new tissue as possible with as few surgeries as possible. Due to limitations of cell and ECM replacement, the current best approaches are total visceral organ transplantation and body transplantation.

Another advantage of body transplants is that they are possible with today's technology. Further work is needed to get to the safety levels appropriate for the clinic, but surgeons already know how to reconnect vasculature, muscle, and other elements, and we have demonstrated spinal cord repair in the special case of surgical transection.

Many lives are already saved each year through organ donation, many of which come from thousands of brain-dead bodies. Under the right circumstances, a portion of those could be used for body donation. All that's needed to begin offering body transplants is for a group to create surgical protocols to ensure high rates of survival and functional recovery.

As we have seen, these natural donors will eventually be replaced by genetically matched human tissue constructs. There are already companies creating tissue constructs that could be used for body transplantation, and others focusing on developing the surgery needed to make use of them. The industry is young, but the work has already begun.

In the meantime, there are more basic replacement therapies that are becoming available that might be good options for some people. The most immediate is replacing your microbiome, with commercial options for rejuvenating oral microbiota, skin microbiota, and others.

Another option worth considering involves your blood. Changing out the oil in your car can have benefits, and there's some evidence that something similar can be done with blood. For example, some groups are offering therapeutic plasma exchange. This therapy replaces some of the fluids in your circulatory system to help remove age-associated signaling molecules and other extracellular junk. It's already on the market, but is less well tested than microbiota transplantation.

Coming up soon will be mitochondrial replacement therapies that could have a big impact both on lifespan and quality of life. Next-gen ECM injectables are also near-horizon, and new cell therapies are coming soon as well. Keep in mind that these approaches are minor in the grand scheme of things, and that big gains will only come from future technology that is not currently available, but hopefully coming soon.

The main thing to remember is that replacement is a conceptually simple solution to aging. It requires almost no understanding of aging, and relatively little understanding of biology. Not only is replacement an efficient strategy, it's also incredibly effective—so effective that it will not only solve some aspects of aging and age-related disease, but many unrelated diseases as well.

Of course, it's a big engineering challenge to produce large supplies of replacement components and deliver them safely at scale. However, many of these obstacles are well understood, and the time until they are solved is merely a matter of money and effort. So lend a hand, and seize this unique opportunity to strike a mortal blow against aging.

Replacement may be the fastest path to radical life extension, but it isn't the only one. The most graceful approach would be to take control of our biology and rewrite it directly.

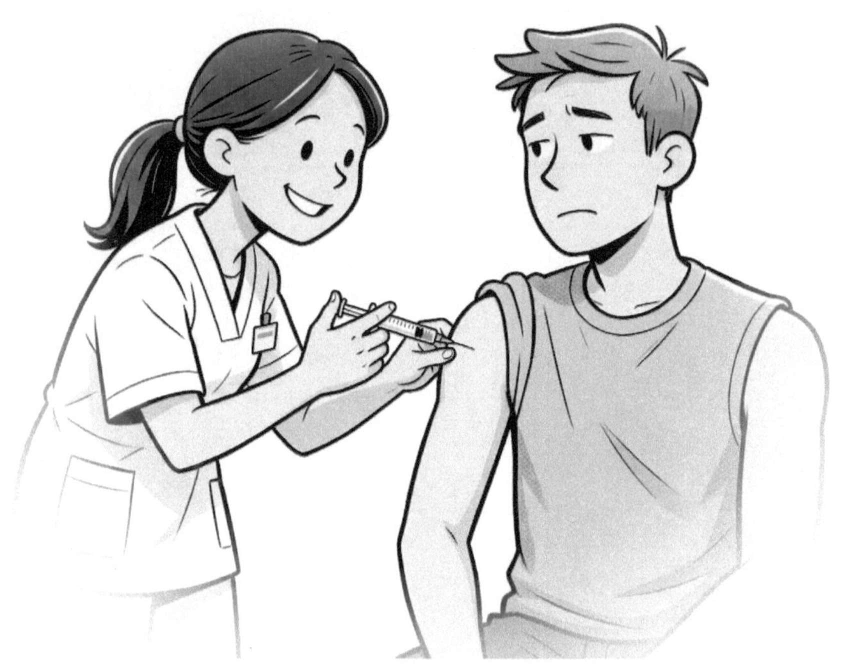

CHAPTER 8

BIOENGINEERING

A bioengineering solution to aging would mean that everyone could simply receive an injection to change their DNA in a way that keeps them young and healthy forever. While that's currently impossible, bioengineering holds enormous potential for curing diseases and radically extending lifespans. It applies scientific and engineering techniques from many disciplines to alter human biology. Like replacement, it could be a complete solution to aging.

Modern bioengineering tools have grown quite powerful and scalable. So powerful, in fact, that we don't fully understand how to use them. However, there is good reason to expect these approaches will eventually solve the most common causes of death. They have already treated genetic diseases, infectious diseases, cancer, and many others.

Tools

Bioengineers wield a diverse toolkit, ranging from small molecules and antibodies to proteins, RNA, and radioactive isotopes. These tools reach into a cell more powerfully than any pill. They can edit the DNA inside cells, fixing broken genes or adding completely new ones. They can bypass DNA entirely and directly deliver mRNA to cells to change the proteins they produce and secrete. They can alter the epigenetic control of DNA expression, sometimes dramatically changing cell behavior. They can peer into the body with ever-increasing clarity. The list goes on.

Bioengineering has another property that could rapidly advance our ability to treat aging: the digitization of human biology. Cells are like little computers running programs, and we're beginning to understand the language those programs are written in, their inputs, and their outputs. As we develop increasingly accurate models of cells and human systems, we will be able to borrow every tool from information technology to drive progress in bioengineering. If historical trends in computing are any indication, the more biology can be treated as an information system, the more progress will accelerate.

These and other techniques will be useful for enhancing human health and longevity. They will also enable improvement of some aspects of human biology beyond natural levels. This is important for radical life extension because we should not limit our thinking to fixing what is broken. To achieve longevity escape velocity as quickly as possible, we need to opportunistically improve some of our biological functions beyond what would typically be seen in even the healthiest young person and use that extraordinary functionality to compensate for other areas that have not yet been rejuvenated.

Bioengineering has such incredible potential that it's hard to imagine everything that will be possible. Eventually humans may be immune to most pathogens, able to regrow limbs like salamanders, or live for hundreds of years—all because of enhancements made to human biology. Such dramatic changes may take a long time to develop, but there are many smaller improvements that can be made along the way. Some have already been achieved in laboratory settings, and many more are in progress.

Historically, doctors have relied on relatively simple drugs found in nature or designed in a lab. Modern bioengineering therapies engage cells in more powerful ways than traditional pharmaceuticals. For example, it's possible to alter cell behavior by engineering targeted antibodies. These antibodies might attach to receptors to disrupt signaling pathways, or they might attach to molecules outside cells to induce cells to interact with them. Antibodies can also be combined with drugs to form antibody-drug conjugates. These increase the concentration of drugs near the antibody targets, enhancing their effects or allowing for lower drug concentrations to be used. Similarly, bispecific antibodies can help bring different molecules or cells together, catalyzing specific reactions or processes.

Antibodies can be manufactured and given to patients directly, or they can be created inside the patient's body by leveraging the cells' existing gene expression systems.

Another example of a modern technique is DNA editing. It's currently possible to read and rewrite the DNA of a cell, altering which RNAs are produced. This leads to the production of different noncoding RNAs, as well as messenger RNAs that are then translated into proteins. Both types of RNA can significantly affect cell behavior. The technology for reading DNA has improved swiftly over the last two decades, to the point where it's now possible to decode the genome of a single human cell.

One common way DNA is currently read is through sequencing by synthesis. DNA is first isolated from a cell, broken into small pieces with vibrations, and attached to a glass dish containing DNA polymerase, an enzyme that builds DNA strands. After that, color-coded nucleotides are sequentially added to the dish and a camera watches what color is used for each piece of DNA at each time point. So if you see red, green, red, blue in a particular location, you know there's DNA there with a sequence of GCGA. Then a computer program puts all the short sequences in order. For a few hundred dollars, you can now have your genome sequenced in roughly a week.

Rewriting genetic information is more challenging because, unlike reading it, you can't just burst open a cell and see what's inside. You need to make edits while the system is still running. Fortunately, biology has evolved a great deal of machinery for modifying and repairing DNA—machinery that can be harnessed to edit a cell's DNA without hurting the cell.

One of the most powerful techniques currently available is called twin prime editing—in effect, a search-and-replace for the genome. It uses a special protein that can both cut DNA and convert RNA into

DNA, paired with guide RNAs that lock onto the unique gene sequence you want to edit. This technique allows you to add, edit, or delete DNA sequences relatively safely and can currently make changes on the order of hundreds of bases.

It's also currently possible to read and rewrite the epigenetics of a cell. Epigenetic information—the molecular cues that control which genes are expressed—is harder to read than DNA. This is because while DNA is stored in a single format, epigenetic information exists in many forms. Cells can add chemical tags to DNA, modify histone proteins that DNA wraps around, attach regulatory proteins, use chromatin-bound RNA, and alter chromatin shape in 3D space. All of these configurations change which genes are active. The good news is that we now have tools to measure each of these layers.

Reading can be done through different techniques like microarrays, which are fast, and sequencing, which captures more information. To get the current best possible picture of an epigenome, you would need seven different assays to cover all the different types of epigenetic information.

Editing the epigenome is also more difficult than editing the genome for the same reason. Fortunately, there are several powerful tools for doing so, many of which are based on dCas9, a protein that can home in on specific locations in the genome. If you can find the epigenetic switch, it's easier to flip on or off.

There are also technologies that can alter epigenetics in a less targeted way. Small molecule drugs can cause genome-wide methylation or demethylation. Similarly, there are small molecule drugs that can globally increase or decrease the epigenetic marks on histones.

One powerful use of epigenetic editing is to push a cell to become a particular cell type. A cell naturally wants to adopt a certain job, like a muscle cell or a nerve cell. Epigenetic reprogramming can convince a cell to change from one type to another, or even from a somatic cell like a skin cell to a pluripotent stem cell. This can be done with reprogramming factors like transcription factor proteins that directly influence genetic circuits, or with RNAs or small molecules that indirectly cause shifts in gene expression. This is how induced-pluripotent stem cells are created. It's also how partial reprogramming works, where cells are given cues to reset their epigenetic state without changing their cell type.

It's also possible to bypass the genome and epigenome of a cell by directly delivering RNA into cells. This RNA can perform a variety of functions. Messenger RNA, or mRNA, can be delivered to cells to produce proteins. These proteins can then work together to perform ordinary tasks that the cell usually does, or they can have new functions that don't normally exist in human biology. For example, if you design an enzyme that can break down molecular waste, you don't have to produce that enzyme in a factory and then inject it into a person. Instead, you can use their cells as a factory and simply inject the mRNA blueprint. Then the patient's own cells will produce the protein for a little while.

RNA can also indirectly affect the expression of genes and the production of proteins. Small interfering RNA, or siRNA, can inhibit the expression of specific mRNA in the cell, leading to the downregulation of metabolic pathways. RNA can also attach itself to the genome, exerting some epigenetic control over cell behavior.

With all of these tools, the next question is how best to use them.

Applications

Manipulation of the genome and epigenome is an incredibly powerful tool. With control of the genome, you can fix small errors in genes that cause disease. This is already happening for people with diseases like hereditary transthyretin amyloidosis, where a mutation leads to harmful protein aggregation in the heart and other tissues. Not only can broken genes be fixed, but risky genes can be replaced with protective ones. For example, if you happen to have two copies of the best version of the FOXO3 gene, you're likely to live a few years longer than someone with two copies of the worst version. But with gene editing you could change your DNA to have the best version of this and many other genes.

Not only that, but even better versions of many genes could be designed. For example, genes that lead to proteins that are likely to aggregate could be adjusted to make proteins that still do the same job, but don't stick together. Similar improvements could be made to noncoding RNAs.

And while we're designing proteins, why not create entirely new ones? Humans don't have an enzyme to break down certain substances that accumulate in our bodies. But we could design such enzymes, and then add genes to our cells to produce them. For example, this could allow us to break down and clear lipofuscin from our cells.

Often, designing new genes isn't even necessary. There are many genes available in other species that could potentially be copied over to humans to help prevent cancer, resist toxins, and heal wounds.

With control of the epigenome, you could optimize cell function and even radically change an organism's biology. Older people suffer from stem cell exhaustion, where they don't have enough stem cells to maintain sufficient somatic cells to keep their tissues and organs fully populated and functioning. But with epigenetic control, you could turn some somatic cells into stem cells in whatever tissues need them. For instance, the fat cells creeping into the thymus and other organs with advanced age could be converted into the cells that the tissue actually needs.

Random changes occur to both genetics and epigenetics with age, but these could theoretically be fixed as well. Corrections to DNA could help prevent cells from spreading into somatic mosaicism and cancer. Reversing the epigenetic drift that occurs randomly with age could get cells back on target for their intended roles and perhaps make them more resistant to such changes.

If we want radical life extension, we should be open to radical therapies as well, and control of genetics will allow us to make much more drastic changes to our bodies. For example, viruses are dependent on cellular machinery to replicate themselves. They carry their own genetic information and then hijack cells to read it and produce proteins to make more viruses. But this only works because viruses use the same genetic language as our cells. Anytime a human cell wants to add tryptophan to a protein, it uses the sequence "TGG," so anytime a virus wants tryptophan it will use the same sequence. However, we could change the coding of human cells to use different sequences for different amino acids. By altering a person's DNA sequence and, at the same time, altering the code their cells use to make proteins, the cell would produce the same proteins it always had. However, any virus that managed to get into the cell would be unable to replicate, because it would be asking for the wrong amino acids. This would make humans immune to all currently existing viruses and potentially have a profound effect on lifespan.

Another radical change in human biology would be to add the ability to regenerate tissues and organs. In response to injury, adult humans produce a lot of collagen, which turns into scar tissue with limited utility. By contrast, animals like salamanders and zebrafish have an extreme regenerative ability. With these animals, you can cut off a limb and it will grow back. To do this, they produce a softer ECM with developmental cues that allow and induce cells to migrate and rebuild tissue. This response could perhaps be adapted into the human genome to allow not only recovery from injury, but rejuvenation through regeneration.

The idea would be to have regenerative capacity that not only restores what you had before an injury, but constructs replacement tissue that's biologically younger than the original. From the perspective of aging damage, this possibility should not be surprising. As long as freshly constructed ECM is organized properly, it should have much less age-related damage accumulation, like cross-links and extracellular aggregates. Similarly, newly produced cells should have much less lipofuscin and oxidized molecules per cell, as many types of cell damage dilute during cell division. So removing and regenerating tissue is a potential solution for clearing large swaths of aging damage from an organism.

There's even some precedent in humans. Human fetuses can recover from injury without scarring up until 24 weeks of gestation. So if you perform surgery on a young fetus, the surgical site will look normal and healthy by the time the baby is born. Surgeries done after the 24-week mark will produce scars, as in adults. Even adults can regenerate certain tissues. A healthy adult liver can regrow lost portions in two or three months. Adult bones are also able to regenerate to some extent, as are peripheral nerves.

Chopping off limbs wouldn't be very pleasant, but it might not be necessary to get the same benefits. It may be possible to destroy and rebuild certain tissues in a wavefront, only tearing down and regenerating a small section at a time. Or, if that proves to be unfeasible, perhaps a diffuse rebuilding of tissue could happen, where a random 1% of the tissue volume is destroyed and rebuilt. Or maybe there are stranger options, like growing backup organs in your own body. The old ones could shrink and make way as the new ones take over their functions.

We'll see where the science takes us, but we should be open to big ideas. They might not work out, but will help expand our thinking about what can be accomplished with bioengineering. There are probably even more unbelievable things that can be done, but even the first generation of technologies that are currently in development look like they will have a meaningful impact on healthspan and lifespan.

The Design Problem

So will bioengineering lead to radical life extension? Yes, but probably not anytime soon. Advanced bioengineering technology is in its infancy, and the more life-altering and life-extending use cases seem to be far off, because there are some major obstacles to applying bioengineering to ameliorate the effects of aging. The first is that we don't know what changes to make to reverse aging. This is the design problem.

To put the problem in perspective, consider the huge advances in molecular biology since the structure of DNA was discovered in the 1950s. In spite of all the hard work and rapidly advancing science, we currently have a good understanding of only about 20% of the 20,000 protein-coding genes. There are many that we have some basic understanding of, but on the other end of the spectrum there's another 20% we have almost no grasp of. To make things worse, most genes don't even make proteins. They make noncoding RNAs that have their own regulatory or metabolic functions. For nonprotein-coding genes, things are much worse—we understand only a few percent of them.

Worse still, even if we knew what RNAs and proteins were being produced, there are big blind spots in metabolic pathways and cell signaling. We haven't even scratched the surface of gene regulatory networks, protein-protein interactions, let alone any sort of useful simulation of what goes on in a cell. The unknowns in biology dwarf the knowns.

Even assuming we could build a solid understanding of the existing system, it wouldn't be immediately clear what changes to make. We have a few ideas for borrowing cancer suppression genes from large mammals or modifying existing proteins so they are less likely to misfold. However, solving aging will require more than just tweaks. It will require new genetic programming on a massive scale.

For example, this might mean creating thousands of new genes and edits that never existed before. Each would need to not only provide specific anti-aging effects, but also play nicely with every other gene. Creating a single such anti-aging gene is a massive undertaking on its own, which is why most people are focusing on the relatively easy approach of modifying existing genes. Given the effort required for large effect sizes, we're likely a long way from being able to design complete solutions to every type of age-related damage.

Even if we did, there is another technological limitation that stands in the way of a bioengineering solution to aging.

The Delivery Problem

The second major obstacle is that, even if we did know what we wanted to change, we wouldn't be able to make the changes in adults. It's one thing to do a simple genetic change in a single cell. It's quite another thing to make complex edits to all the cells in a human body. This is called the delivery problem.

If human cells were grains of sand, yours would fill an Olympic swimming pool. If you wanted to put a dot of green paint on each grain of sand you could try spraying some paint on top, but then the sand at the bottom of the pool would not get any. You could pour in a lot of paint so that some gets to the bottom, but then the top would get too much. Similarly, doctors can get gene therapies to some cells in the body, but it's hard to get the right amount to every cell.

The delivery problem is harder than that, because drugs delivered to the body don't necessarily go where you want them to go or spread out in an intuitive way. They tend to accumulate in the liver and lungs, and it's especially hard to get drugs into the brain. Even if you can get a therapy to the right tissue, it's challenging to control which cell types will take it up. Assuming you can get a gene therapy into the right cell, there's still the problem of making sure the right amount gets in. Too little and you might not get the therapeutic effect. Too much and you may cause damage. It's hard to get an even delivery across cells within a tissue. If that weren't enough, you still want to ensure that your therapy is activated at the right time and under the right circumstances, such as at the right phase of the cell cycle or during the appropriate epigenetic state.

Even if you get the right amount into a cell, gene therapies might have unintended consequences, for example off-target effects that cause unwanted genetic or epigenetic changes. So, while we have good tools for editing cells in a dish, delivering gene therapies in living bodies remains an unsolved problem.

We're left with the dual problems of not knowing what changes to make to solve aging with bioengineering nor how to deliver them even if we did. So any strategy for radical life extension that heavily relies on bioengineering must address these problems as prerequisites. These are both active areas of development, with many scientists trying to build solutions.

Delivery Strategies

Currently, the main options for delivering gene therapies in people include viruses, lipid nanoparticles, and proteolipid vehicles. These each take a payload of RNA or DNA and deliver it into cells.

Viruses are normally dangerous because they carry genetic instructions to produce more viruses. However, scientists found a way to remove viral instructions and replace them with gene therapies. These modified viruses float around until they find a cell to infect and inject their cargo, but the new medicinal cargo makes you healthier rather than sick.

Two common viruses used for gene therapies are adeno-associated virus and lentiviral vectors. Viral vectors are relatively easy to produce and different strains have evolved affinities for specific cell types, a feature that can be very useful. Unfortunately, viral vectors often trigger an immune response that can sometimes be fatal. Some can only be used once before the body develops antibodies against them, and some people already have these antibodies before they even get their first gene therapy.

Lipid nanoparticles (LNPs) are spherical particles that hold DNA or RNA inside a synthetic lipid membrane. They are structurally simple, relatively easy to manufacture, and have low immunogenicity. When injected into the body, cells ingest them via endocytosis, and then they can occasionally break free and release their contents into the cell's cytosol. They are typically not very efficient, with most of the LNPs going to the liver, and most LNPs that get inside cells getting broken down in lysosomes.

Proteolipid vehicles are similar to lipid nanoparticles, except that they have special fusion proteins on their surface. This allows them to fuse with a cell membrane and dump their contents in directly. This makes them more efficient in delivering payloads. By tailoring the surface proteins to have affinities for certain cell types, some control of distribution across tissues and cell types has been achieved. So proteolipid vehicles have the good distribution and efficient delivery of viruses but the low immunogenicity of LNPs. While this is a big improvement, there is still much work to do on improving delivery.

Another strategy is to try to develop therapies that don't need targeted delivery. For example, you can focus on gene therapies that are effective wherever they happen to go. These treatments can work locally but act globally, usually by causing cells to secrete signaling molecules. This is how certain mRNA vaccines work.

If you just want to turn some cells into little factories for circulating molecules, that isn't too difficult to do with today's technology. For example, you can inject a gene therapy into a group of fat cells that will cause them to produce the protein Klotho, which has been shown to improve lifespan in animals. Other things that might be effective include adiponectin, an anti-inflammatory protein that centenarians often have high levels of, exercise mimetics like irisin and MOTS-c, and brain-derived neurotrophic factor, which seems to have protective effects in the brain.

Exercise mimetics are particularly interesting because top athletes have an exceptionally low incidence of many diseases, including heart disease. If the body could be programmed to react to a gene therapy the way it reacts to high levels of exercise, then a variety of diseases of aging could be delayed, extending healthspan and lifespan. Complete exercise mimetic drugs don't yet exist, but bioengineers have some partial results. For example, there are gene therapies that can cause muscles to grow, and using these might compensate for sarcopenia and its symptoms while waiting for the underlying cause to be fully resolved.

Another path forward exploits the fact that delivery vectors tend to go to the liver by developing therapies for liver-related diseases. For example, there are gene therapies for hemophilia A and B that fix the problem by introducing normal genes into liver cells. Another is the siRNA therapy inclisiran, which modifies the metabolism of lipids by your liver in a way that reduces cardiovascular disease risk.

Because of the relative ease of delivery, the lungs are another area that might benefit from early gene therapies. Current therapies targeting the lungs include clinical trials for cystic fibrosis and idiopathic pulmonary fibrosis, among others. Similarly, the skin is eminently targetable, with approved and in-clinical-trial gene therapies for dystrophic epidermolysis bullosa, melanoma, and more.

One clever way to mitigate the delivery problem is to develop gene therapies that are only activated when they are in the right context. For example, companies are developing programmable mRNA therapies that can activate or deactivate depending on cell type and state. This would make delivery easier because you could use a nonspecific delivery mechanism that got the therapy to many cells, but would only affect the cells you're targeting.

This programmability is useful in other ways as well. You can theoretically build new gene circuits, which are the biological feedback loops that allow genes to influence the expression of other genes. Gene circuits are like smoke detectors—if they sense trouble they can set off the fire alarm or even the sprinkler system—this is termed "negative feedback" and is a crucial mechanism for cells to maintain a healthy state. Just like a smart home, a cell has many smart systems, like gene circuit thermostats, security alarms, and so on. With the right gene circuits, you could control how much work a specific therapy does in a given cell. So for example, even if a cell receives multiple deliveries of a gene therapy that makes protein X, the negative feedback circuit could ensure that only the desired amount of protein X is produced. This could help mitigate the problem of uneven distribution of gene delivery.

Yet another strategy for getting around the delivery problem is to reprogram cells ex vivo. Simply take the cells out of a person's body, make the edits to the cells in a laboratory setting, and then put the cells back in. Of course, cells suffer from their own delivery problems, but there are benefits to this approach. The first is that ex vivo techniques for getting therapies into cells are much more effective and widely available. Second, quality control can be done on the cells before they are reintroduced, ensuring that the therapy did what it was supposed to, and nothing else. If you want to update cells that are just floating around the circulatory system, like immune cells, then this is a great approach.

This technique has been used in several treatments already on the market. One of the most common is CAR-T cell therapy, where immune cells are modified to produce special receptors on their surface. This causes them to attack specific targets, like leukemias. Many groups are now working on ways to add the chimeric antigen receptors in vivo by delivering gene therapies to the T cells without removing them first. regulatory T cells can also be modified to help suppress autoimmune disease and to fight cancer.

Another potential use of cells is to take somatic cells from a patient, induce pluripotency, and then differentiate the cells before returning them to the patient to treat conditions like macular degeneration, Parkinson's disease, and heart failure.

These are all great approaches, but cells that are reprogrammed ex vivo could potentially do a lot more. Cells could be used to deliver therapies where they need to go, using their natural homing abilities, or new ones that could be programmed in. They could be programmed to remove built-up debris like amyloids, or clear senescent cells. Cells could be used in more intelligent cancer suppression, or to restore healthy signaling in fluids and reduce inflammation. They could be sent in to help rebuild the network of blood vessels throughout the body, improving blood flow and tissue function. Reprogrammed cells could also be used to protect the body from autoimmune diseases and avoid rejection of transplanted organs. They might even be able to help rebuild the ECM throughout the body, replacing worn-out proteins with young, healthy ones. Or, as a first step, they could help remove some of the damaged ECM to make way for natural turnover.

One idea for actually solving the delivery problem is to use a somatic gene drive. A gene drive is a gene therapy that can install instructions for a cell to make and secrete new copies of the gene drive. Like a virus, these copies could then go into other cells that would produce more copies, eventually spreading the update to all cells in the body. Various therapeutic payloads can be installed along with the gene drive, and these would spread across cells exponentially. You would want the gene drive to be designed to only install once inside any particular cell, and also have some limit on how long it would actively produce copies, which are additional engineering challenges. However, with proper safeguards, this could conceptually allow for easy, systemic delivery of gene therapies and overcome one major hurdle for bioengineering.

The biggest benefit to solving the delivery problem wouldn't be any immediate improvement in functionality, but the ability to edit a body to make future updates easier and more reliable. You could have your first change install a genetic mechanism to facilitate delivery of future updates into the cells; making it easy to deliver new edits over time, all while reducing the risks associated with current approaches to gene delivery: toxicity, off-target effects, immunogenicity, small payload size, and poor distribution.

Right now we have trouble delivering gene therapies, so we should take every opportunity to make that easier. We can do so by making strategic changes to our DNA that make it safer and easier to insert new genes, as well as making sure that the appropriate number of changes are made. Creating a sort of update platform would allow for safe, easy, and repeatable insertion of new DNA. It could be designed to allow only a single such insertion per gene therapy in any given cell. This would be something like a genetic landing pad with a unique sequence. Each time a new insertion was made, that insertion would update the landing sequence to something different, so that additional copies of the gene therapy would not insert themselves, but future therapies could target the new sequence.

If you happen not to be born yet, then the easiest way around the delivery problem would be to have your parents genetically modify their gametes before conceiving you, and you would benefit from all the fixes. Or, if you're recently conceived, current technology can deliver the edits to you directly while you are a zygote or embryo. While the ethics of this are still being worked out, these delivery methods could become one of the most impactful ways to reduce suffering around the world.

Targeting Damage

If we want radical life extension through bioengineering, we'll need to tackle the different types of age-related damage.

One type of damage we need to contend with is the accumulation of problematic molecules inside cells. These are mostly metabolic byproducts of normal chemical reactions, none of which are perfectly efficient, though some are pollutants you absorbed from the environment. A common form of this damage is called lipofuscin, which is a mix of lipids, proteins, and metals that build up in lysosomes either because they are resistant to digestion or because some other damage is interfering with the lysosome's digestive abilities. Others include proteins like alpha-synuclein that can end up folded improperly, leading to aggregation inside cells, or oxidized cholesterol derivatives that are hard for cells to break down, and old proteins that are marked for degradation but somehow avoided being cleared.

Here the work required is to develop proteins that can break down these problematic molecules or package them for removal and excretion. Our cells could then be made to manufacture those proteins via DNA edits or periodic mRNA therapies.

Accumulation of this type of damage could probably be slowed greatly if proteins were modified to make them less likely to misfold and easier to correct when they do. Proteins that aggregate could be changed to reduce the chances of them clumping together, like alpha-synuclein. Similarly, prion and prion-like proteins could be changed to avoid their harmful propagation.

One of the hardest types of damage to resolve with bioengineering is likely to be DNA mutations. Though we have the technology to edit DNA, there's a lot of DNA in the human body, and random changes anywhere can lead to cancer, or less dangerous gangs of mutated cells as seen in clonal expansion.

We don't need to solve the general problem of DNA mutations to make progress. Much easier would be to first correct all single-point mutations you inherited, restoring proper function of genes. To do that, a sample of your cells needs to be sequenced, then guide RNAs can be synthesized and combined with gene editing enzymes to repair those mutations. Genes could also be updated to their longevity-promoting alleles, such as the APOE2 variant, which strongly reduces Alzheimer's risk.

However, fixing random DNA mutations accumulated with age is much harder. Imagine your local library was shrunk to the size of a poppy seed, and you had to check each minuscule book for typos. That doesn't break the laws of physics, but it's hard to imagine in the foreseeable future. In the near term, we can likely improve DNA repair mechanisms to slow DNA damage accumulation and clear cells with particularly dangerous mutations.

Epigenetic drift is currently difficult to solve for the same reason. Random changes happen across a very large number of possible epigenetic states. In addition, the relative transience of the epigenome could make it harder to achieve complete rejuvenation if corrected in small portions at a time. Unlike DNA edits that can be expected to be durable, one round of epigenetic edits might be undone before the next round of changes is made.

Fortunately, human cells seem to have an innate ability to undo random epigenetic damage. Just as an experienced musician will know if a certain note doesn't sound right in a song, a cell can sometimes tell if epigenetic switches are in the wrong position and flip them back. Companies are currently developing tools to build on this innate epigenetic reprogramming for cellular rejuvenation. If successful, there could be a single therapy that resets a large amount of random changes, greatly reducing the scope of the problem.

If we could solve all epigenetic and genetic mutations, we wouldn't have to worry about cancer. That is a long way off, so it makes sense to spend time developing different therapies against it. We could add additional genes to protect against cancer. Ideas include inserting extra copies of the p53 tumor suppressor gene, as is seen in large mammals like elephants. Similarly, adding extra copies of the PTEN gene could help; engineered mice with elevated PTEN are strongly resistant to cancer. Naked mole rats take a different approach, producing more and larger versions of the ECM component hyaluronan, which helps suppress cancer by physically restraining cells. Whales have superior DNA repair machinery that would be nice to have, too.

Somatic mosaicism would also be resolved with complete rejuvenation of genetic and epigenetic mutations. Ahead of that, it's probably possible to identify cells that have mutated to out-compete their peers and correct the problem. This could be done by editing away the mutations, clearing the cells, or introducing superior qualities to healthy cells to eventually outcompete the ones that are causing trouble.

Sometimes mutations aren't the problem, but the solution. For example, the transposable elements in our DNA can cause DNA damage as epigenetic suppression of them is lost at older ages. But if you intentionally mutate them so they can't reactivate, then you also stop them from damaging your DNA.

Senescent cells can also be created via DNA damage or other types of damage. Many companies are working on approaches to mitigate problems caused by senescent cells, with senolytics that kill them outright, senomorphics that reverse senescence, or therapies that prevent senescence in the first place. Clearing seems the safest and most straightforward approach because of the potential downsides of interfering with the natural senescence process, but time will tell whether any of these methods are useful.

Clearing might also be the best strategy for certain types of fat cells. You could probably kill large quantities of deep belly fat, known as visceral fat, to reduce inflammation. This could give a nice boost to both healthspan and lifespan. You could also convert white fat, which likes to store energy, to brown fat, which likes to burn energy, and reap some additional metabolic benefits. Fat isn't all bad, so encouraging it to return to the locations and quantities of youth will not only make you feel better, but also protect your body.

Another contender for hardest problem to solve is extracellular matrix damage. Imagine how hard it would be to take a fried egg and restore it to its raw state. To some extent, your ECM gets cooked over the course of your life, and cells don't know how to fix it. Any therapy that rejuvenates the ECM would need to not only ensure the production of young, high-quality ECM but also the correct composition of ECM for each individual tissue. What's more, the structure and geometry of the ECM need to be correct for each tissue as well. So putting the right building blocks together in the wrong way, or the wrong ones in the right way, will lead to dysfunctional tissue rather than rejuvenation.

It's not just about rebuilding ECM, though. You also need to clear away the old ECM. That's not trivial, as ECM molecules accumulate strong chemical cross-links over time. These links make the ECM dense and difficult for degrading enzymes and molecules to penetrate, so simple strategies like upregulating the production of ECM-degrading proteins like matrix metalloproteases will only make things worse, as this only hastens the destruction of young ECM and leaves old ECM unscathed.

In addition to repairing the ECM itself, protein aggregates and plaques that build up in the ECM would need to be cleared. These can disrupt tissue function, leading to poor organ performance. For example, transthyretin can cause amyloid cardiomyopathy, where protein aggregates into amyloid fibrils that are hard for the body to break down. The buildup of protein in the heart can stiffen it and lead to heart failure.

It has been demonstrated that protein aggregates can be cleared with antibodies and with enzymes, so there's a path forward to creating therapies for this kind of aging damage. Once the appropriate proteins are designed, genes to produce them can be delivered to our cells to manufacture them as needed.

Not only does the quality of ECM degrade as we age, but the macrostructure also changes in harmful ways. The spine can shrink and curve with age. Vasculature weakens and bulges into conditions like varicose veins. It isn't enough to clear away junk and replace the existing molecules. The original structure of the tissue needs to be reconstituted to fully rejuvenate the body. Cells have some innate knowledge of what size and shape tissues and organs should be, so it should be possible to direct them to do the reconstruction. How to do that effectively is an open question.

Another ECM-related problem is excess bone growth. Many people suffer from bone density loss, but there are other conditions like Paget's disease where too much bone is produced. Researchers have also found that age-related bone growth can narrow the drainage channels leading out of the skull, reducing the outflow of cerebrospinal fluid into the body. Since this fluid carries away waste products, it has been proposed that the resulting buildup contributes to neurodegeneration. Some companies are looking at ways of physically restoring outflow of CSF, and it should be possible to develop gene therapies that solve this problem as well.

ECM damage also interferes with stem cell niches, leading to stem cell exhaustion, which then leads to loss of cell populations; this is a hallmark of aging, causing tissue function to decline as the supply of replacement somatic cells decreases. It's hard to maintain muscle mass without stem cells to provide the material. But stem cells would last much longer if various types of damage were repaired. Young ECM has been shown to improve cell behavior, so rejuvenating the ECM might be sufficient to keep stem cells working long enough for longevity escape velocity. Or we might need to fix several types of damage to maintain healthy cell populations.

Mitochondrial dysfunction should also be solvable with gene therapies. Mitochondria are kept in large quantities in each cell, have their own small genomes called mtDNA, and they can be rebuilt and recycled. A major cause of their dysfunction is mutations to the mtDNA, some of which gain a selective advantage causing them to displace healthy mitochondria. Conceptually, we could use bioengineering to keep mitochondrial populations healthy and productive just by periodically clearing out the old mutated mtDNA and replacing it with new copies. Perhaps even include some upgrades to make them more resistant to damage or better at producing energy.

Enhancements

So far, we've played defense, repairing damage. But we can also go on offense, adding new qualities to our cells and tissues. What we think of as damage is a detrimental change away from normal, whereas beneficial changes away from normal are enhancements. The accumulation of these upgrades will probably be a part of many paths to radical life extension.

For example, what if we designed new, improved DNA repair mechanisms? Slowing the rate of mutations would extend healthspan and lifespan, and there might be secondary benefits as well, such as resistance to radiation. That's not just helpful when your dentist takes x-rays of your teeth, but also when you fly in a plane or eat a banana.

Even if your DNA is perfect, age-related problems can occur with the fundamental processes of transcription and translation. So, enhancements to the core machinery of RNA and protein production could slow the rate of aging and delay age-related decline.

It may be helpful to add or remove the ability to internally produce certain vitamins or amino acids. Adding means we would no longer be dependent on getting them from our diet. On the other hand, removing or reducing production of things that are now easy to get through diet could be a net benefit by lessening the work your body needs to do, which could lead to slower damage accumulation.

Another area for improvement is to remove the late-life costs of genes that are helpful during development, but detrimental later in life, a phenomenon known as antagonistic pleiotropy. Some of these evolved because of advantages conveyed in our ancestral environment, but are no longer relevant. Consider a gene that makes you more likely to reproduce, but also more likely to get diabetes later in life. Evolution would favor it, but we could make ourselves healthier by deactivating it in middle age.

While it may be easy to come up with ideas for things to change, human biology has limitations that will make certain plausible-sounding changes undesirable due to negative trade-offs. You may say you want to be as strong as a bear, but the muscles that are good for strength aren't necessarily good for endurance and fine motor control. You may be able to open any jar in the kitchen with your bare hands, but then you might have a hard time using chopsticks.

Even so, straight improvements are possible, and we should not be discouraged just because we have to work within some constraints. There are likely to be protein designs that are just better than their normal counterparts. Imagine enzymes that do their work 10 or 100 times faster, or are smaller and easier to produce and always fold correctly. You couldn't just install these blindly and expect things to end well, but they could be important options as part of a larger plan for solving aging.

Another area where gains could be made is gut microbiota. Currently we have a mix of helpful and harmful species in our digestive tract. With some work, we could engineer microbes that are even more eager to please, and maybe also help clear out the bad ones.

Perhaps we could induce cells to produce novel anti-infectives that improve upon the body's innate immune system. As discussed earlier, it seems possible to make human cells immune to viruses by changing our genetic code, but viruses aren't the only pathogens we have to contend with. Teaching the body how to take down bacteria, fungi, and other foreign invaders might be just as helpful.

In addition to improving molecular designs, tissues and anatomy could also be optimized. For example, small changes in shape might make your heart last longer or protect your lungs from pollution. Maybe add a second liver, pancreas, or heart, so the failure of one is not so devastating. Perhaps entirely new organs could be designed.

Using comparative biology to look for improvements in other animals has inspired ideas for fighting cancer, but there may be other improvements to be found in long-lived species such as the Greenland shark. There are probably other useful biological tools in short-lived species as well, such as the radiation resistance of extremophiles like tardigrades. Various reptiles have extreme immune systems that allow them to eat a disease-ridden diet. Not that you would do so intentionally, but it would be nice to be immune to food poisoning.

Gene Circuits

As we make our way to becoming genetically modified organisms, we will have to step carefully at first. Most of the changes we would want to make would alter a complex web of metabolic pathways. These pathways are controlled by our genes through gene circuits, the feedback loops that allow cells to adapt to changing conditions.

As our understanding improves, we may be able to program gene circuits more directly—more like software engineering than traditional drug development. By introducing new gene circuits and influencing existing ones, we could control cells in complex ways to achieve outcomes that were impossible with small molecules or simpler gene therapies that merely nudge one metabolic pathway. We could give cells full behavioral programs: detect damage, respond, repair, and stand down. For example, we might be able to design cell types whose job is to find damaged cells, clear them, and replace them.

The power of gene circuits is hard to overstate. It is possible to design gene circuits that detect the runaway growth of cancer and self-destruct the cell before it ever spreads. Cancer might try to mutate its way around this defense, in the same way it happens with our natural anti-cancer machinery. However, with each additional anti-cancer mechanism, the chances of a cell evading them all become statistically much lower.

Not only could gene circuits add new anti-cancer programs to our DNA, but they can potentially be used to alleviate every aspect of aging. Just like cancer, there could be self-destruct timers for senescent cells. Similarly, you could build programs that more robustly recycle mitochondria, and selectively degrade mutated ones to help keep the population healthy. In the same way, genetic software to more intelligently activate autophagy or exocytosis could help cells digest or get rid of internal damage.

Gene circuits will also provide a window into intercellular communication networks. When you understand the program running in a cell, it's easier to decipher the messages coming and going throughout the body. Not only that, but you can design new messages and receivers that protect and improve tissue function.

During development, your body is capable of crafting the exquisite details of your various tissues. In adulthood, many of these programs are no longer useful or can even be detrimental. But with control of gene circuits, we could adapt them to do useful work in adults, such as regrowing lost limbs or cyclically breaking down and regenerating your tissues. In some cases like the lungs and vasculature, it may be easier to program parts to die off and regrow rather than trying to repair them in place. This would allow genetic programmers to reuse existing developmental programs, but could be challenging in organs with low reserve capacity, like the heart. Similarly, it might be easier to program cells to search out ECM cross-links and slowly renovate tissue en masse rather than trying to develop enzymes that can fix each type of damage.

There are many more ways gene circuits could have a big impact. Cellular function could be buttressed. Somatic cells could be made less likely to drift away from their cell type. Stem cells could be programmed to better maintain their niches.

Specialized damage-repair cells might have a single job that they do well, such as removing old ECM components and laying down new ones in the vasculature—the slow, coordinated ECM-rebuilding we saw earlier, but carried out by purpose-built cells. With the ability to program cells like computers, things that were previously impossible will become merely very difficult.

The interconnectedness of human biology would make gene circuit programming difficult for a human to design, but computer programs could be used to identify opportunities for improvement, help design changes, test, and implement them. All of this depends on finding ways to generate models of cells and their interactions. It isn't clear when we will have the data and computational power to do these things. However, when they arrive they should accelerate bioengineering immensely.

Unknown Unknowns

Unlike biostasis and replacement, which have clear paths to achieve their goals, there's no clear plan for bioengineering. There's no technology roadmap that we can march along, or even a sketch that will help us predict what will happen and how long it will take. We will need to take small steps toward a complete solution, learning as we go, until there's sufficient scientific knowledge and technological infrastructure to unleash radical changes to human metabolism. No one can predict how long that will take.

Having said that, it's useful to imagine potential paths toward complete genetic control and estimate when they might arrive. Predictions often go wrong, but there are pressing questions about where to allocate time and resources that can be more effectively addressed if we have some idea about what we might get from pursuing bioengineering technology.

What might a bioengineering solution to longevity look like? Solve the delivery problem, solve the design problem, and train accurate predictive computer models. Then modify the body to crush the top causes of death: no more cardiovascular disease, no more cancer, no more viruses, rejuvenate cell populations, repair DNA, and rebuild the ECM somehow.

Some companies today seem to have promising delivery technology, such as fusion-associated small transmembrane proteins. Other companies have strategies for selective expression of gene therapies based on, for instance, the transcriptome of the cell it is delivered to. So, for the sake of argument, let's assume that selective and even delivery or activation is solved in the next decade.

Even with delivery solved, the prospects for overcoming age-related changes to cells using bioengineering are quite poor. Anything in a cell can be damaged. Cells in vitro can escape from this problem by diluting damage through cell division, but it would be challenging to make use of this mechanism in an adult body. Even if that were made to work, there's still the unsolved problem of mutations. Neither the general accumulation of cell damage nor mutations are anywhere near being solved, but let's generously guess 25 years for bioengineering solutions that program cells to eject damage and completely refresh the genome from time to time.

Even with cellular damage under control, aging ECM will still kill you as the mechanical properties of tissues drift away from what is needed to sustain life. Unfortunately, the prospects for overcoming age-related changes to the extracellular matrix are even less promising.

Whereas cells have direct control of their internal environment, they only have indirect control of their external environment. It's a bit like an air traffic controller talking a passenger through landing a plane.

To make matters worse, the ECM has a strong influence over cell behavior, so the more damaged the ECM, the more work it will be to make cells that can operate effectively inside it. So the passenger trying to land the plane might be screaming in the ear of the air traffic controller. The challenge could be an order of magnitude harder than repairing cells, but let's guess it's merely twice as hard and is completed in 50 years. That's a rosy scenario for young children, but what about everyone else?

With estimates for a complete bioengineering solution to aging ranging from 25 to 100 years, things may seem grim. However, there will be phases of progress, where simple gene therapies begin to solve a few specific issues, making people a little healthier and a little longer-lived. Then perhaps we will see everyone benefiting from optimized genomes with the most protective variants of each gene, and a few newly designed enhancements, making it so that it is more common to live to at least 100 years. At some point, we'll figure out how to repair ECM and keep the brain healthy, and the current upper limits for human lifespan will be broken. This gradual but accelerating progress means that by progressively buying more time, more people will survive to see a full solution to aging than might be expected. There are other limits to lifespan of course, such as accidents and meteors, but they are not worth worrying about until the problem of aging is solved.

Despite huge challenges to overcome, bioengineering offers real promise for life extension. Gene delivery is the breakthrough to watch, and should be a focus for the field. So incorporate bioengineering techniques into your strategy as they arrive—because the payoffs are real: viral immunity could give a big boost, and ECM repair alone could add decades to your life.

Depending on your level of risk tolerance and your doctor's advice, you may want to wait for general availability of a particular therapy after it goes through a number of clinical trials for safety and effectiveness. Or, you may want to go somewhere that offers the medicines after passing only a safety trial, which could get you access to a therapy many years sooner. The extra years spent in relatively good health could be the difference between life and death.

Helping with Biostasis and Replacement

Even if bioengineering will eventually be a complete solution to the problem of aging, it isn't clear how much time and attention the longevity community should spend on it today. If we want to save as many lives as possible, we need to allocate every minute and every dollar to the highest impact projects. Given the enormous efforts already going into bioengineering from the rest of the biotech community, the longevity community might be more effective through limiting bioengineering efforts to a small, selective set of projects. For example, it might make sense to focus bioengineering efforts on opportunities to improve biostasis and replacement.

Perhaps one of the best uses of bioengineering in the short term would be to improve the quality of cryopreservation. The reason is that bioengineering is well situated to greatly improve biostasis, because preservation is a one-time event, so existing, short-lived technologies like mRNA therapy might be used to prepare a patient and greatly improve their preservation quality.

One of the most important tissues for preservation is the vasculature, which is relatively easy to affect with gene therapies. Bioengineering solutions that optimize the vasculature for the preservation process would make the process safer and easier to perform.

Gene therapies could be developed to prepare the brain for preservation. Cells in the brain could be modified to produce protective factors to prevent ice formation themselves, rather than trying to perfuse them in from the outside. Similarly, they could be modified to be more robust against damage from dehydration and mechanical stress. These might be factors that inhibit ice growth or prime the cell to repair itself when rewarmed after the preservation. By using bioengineering approaches, we can help to ensure that the delicate ultrastructure of the brain is preserved as well as possible. Ways of reducing the toxicity of cryoprotectants would also go a long way to improving cryopreservation, and gene therapies could help reduce the trade-off between toxicity and cryoprotection.

After biostasis, the next best use of bioengineering might be to develop better ways to produce replacement tissues and organs. Cell replacement approaches will benefit from tools to improve cell quality, expand cell populations, and modify cell behavior. The production of tissues will benefit from the same, as well as ways of producing more naturally organized and structured tissue. But perhaps the biggest impact that bioengineering will have in the short term is the modification of the developmental processes to allow us to produce human organs and tissues at scale.

Bioengineering will help produce human tissue constructs, make it easier to grow them to size, and make it easier to maintain and keep them healthy until they are needed. Additionally, bioengineering will hopefully help find ways to accelerate the growth and development of replacement parts without compromising their quality and usefulness when they reach the appropriate size.

Bioengineering can also help by ensuring that replacement parts don't elicit or generate an immune response. It would be much cheaper and easier to have a single version of a replacement part that could be used for everyone, rather than growing genetically suitable parts for each patient. The trouble is that you don't want a patient's immune system to reject the part. Or in cases where the replaced tissue contains immune cells, you don't want the replacement immune system attacking the patient. Bioengineering has a number of strategies for avoiding this infighting, and it will be important to continue to improve them so that we can have off-the-shelf replacement parts without immune response and without increasing the risk of cancer.

Bioengineering can also help with the delivery of replacement parts. Therapies that promote repair of tissue damaged during surgery will improve survival and recovery rates. Ways of preparing tissue for faster recovery from injury would be especially advantageous for large-scale replacements like limbs, multivisceral organ transplants, and bodies. Even simple things like getting different tissues to temporarily produce colors that help distinguish them during surgery would be useful.

Helping to accelerate replacement therapies might even be the fastest way to get bioengineering therapies to people. Even if bioengineering can't solve the delivery problem directly, it can still deliver benefits through pre-engineered replacement cells and organs. Anytime you put in something new, make sure it has all the latest genetic enhancements. And if those upgraded parts are easier to deliver gene therapies to, all the better.

Bioengineering may also be essential for repairing the brain. If surgical replacement proves very challenging or even untenable on its own, we may be able to overcome limitations with complementary bioengineering strategies. Perhaps growing new, healthy vasculature and rebuilding neural circuitry in place, or modifying transplants to be able to integrate more effectively with the host brain. This will be a real challenge, but it is one that bioengineers will eventually be up to.

Key Takeaways

Bioengineering may be the future of longevity, but nobody knows when that future will arrive. Cancer is not the hardest problem in longevity, and we are not even close to solving it, let alone all the aspects of aging. Even so, bioengineering has the most money and resources of any part of the longevity field. So while it currently looks like it will take a long time to get a bioengineering solution to aging, there are likely to be some pleasant surprises along the way. People tend to overestimate near-term progress and underestimate long-term progress, so maybe we'll get significant bioengineering breakthroughs in the next few decades. The last few certainly saw major unpredicted advances, such as PCR and CRISPR.

Regardless of how long a complete solution takes, it seems likely that bioengineering fixes and enhancements will allow many people to add years to their healthspan and lifespan. Exciting new therapies are in development, and biotech companies continue to march on. There are gene therapies coming soon that could largely solve cholesterol-related diseases like atherosclerosis. Other treatments seem to permanently protect against certain types of cancer. Not to mention the fat-busting, skin-restoring, and hair-growing therapies that will likely hit the market.

Exciting progress is being made, and soon longevity will get a real shot in the arm. But if you don't have time to wait, there is something you can do right now that will buy you more time than all the currently available bioengineering technology combined. Even better, it is completely free.

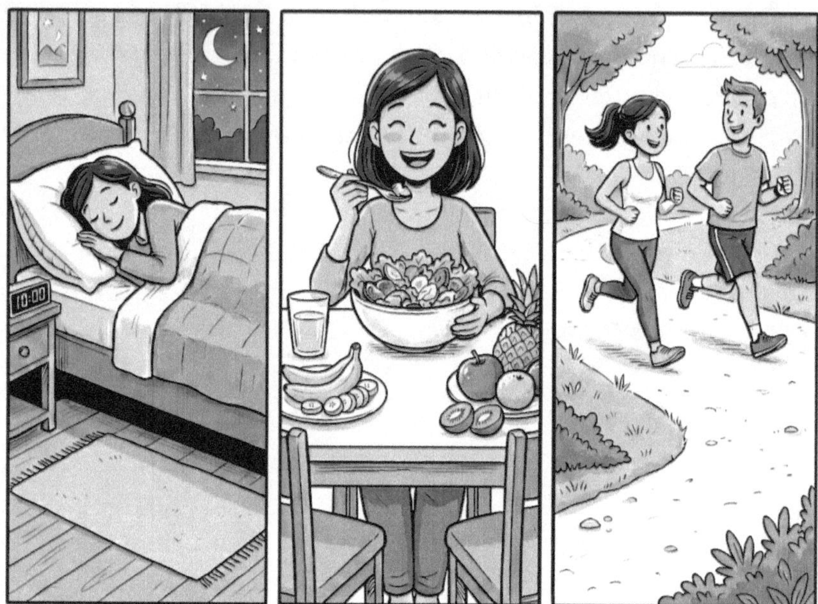

CHAPTER 9

HEALTHY CHOICES

Living a healthy life won't save you, but it will improve your chances of being saved by technology. If you refrain from smoking, you will probably live an extra 10 years compared to someone who does. Ten years is a long time for new technology to develop and for you to put yourself in a better position to benefit from it.

A variety of lifestyle interventions have shown meaningful improvements in health and longevity. We know this because we can see the impact of different lifestyles across a wide variety of human cultures. Switching from an unhealthy diet like the standard American diet or an Eastern European diet to a healthier one, like the traditional Okinawan or Seventh-day Adventist diet, can add years to your life. As part of an overall healthy lifestyle, the gain can approach a decade. Similarly, switching from a sedentary lifestyle to one full of exercise can add several years to your life. That can take you pretty far into the future, so the good news is that developing healthy habits can significantly increase your chances of reaching longevity escape velocity.

Sleep, emotional health, and where you choose to live matter too. Unfortunately, eating well, exercising, and generally taking good care of yourself are simple but not easy. It takes a lot of mental effort and willpower to do what is good for you in the long run, rather than what is easy in the short term. This means that focusing too much on lifestyle optimization can lead to ego depletion, leaving you without the energy to invest in other things that may be equally or more important.

Even within lifestyle optimization, you need to choose wisely how much to focus on each area. You could spend all of your time and money improving your diet, but if you already eat well, you would get more benefit by focusing on sleep and exercise instead. More importantly, even if you strike the right balance among sleep, exercise, diet, and other lifestyle factors, you still need to make sure you're optimizing lifestyle as a whole against activities that can actually radically extend your lifespan, like helping to push forward longevity technology.

Lifestyle should not be your sole focus and, depending on your personal circumstances, perhaps not even your primary one. But for most people, it makes sense to spend some time understanding what the ideal lifestyle factors are for maximizing longevity so that they can decide how much to work on each one. Some people like to take the 80/20 approach. With many things in life, you can get 80% of the benefit for 20% of the effort. For example, if you never exercise, but then you start exercising for 30 minutes a day, it will have a much bigger benefit than if you already exercise 90 minutes each day and you bump that up to two hours. Similarly, if you have obvious sleep or diet issues, there might be low-hanging fruit for improving your health.

Another common mistake is getting excited about supplements. Supplements can be useful under two conditions. The first is that you have a deficit of something. Eating food is good for you when you have a calorie deficit, but not so good for you when you have already eaten enough food to maintain a healthy body weight. Similarly, a dietary supplement can be useful if you're deficient in a particular vitamin or mineral. For example, people who live near the North or South Pole go through periods with very little sunlight, so it's hard for them to manufacture enough vitamin D. So, for them, and for people who spend a lot of time indoors, it makes sense to take a supplement.

Another factor is that a supplement must actually do what you think it does. Many supplements don't contain what they claim to contain and, even when they do, the ingredients often don't have the effects people expect. For example, some people believe that taking beta-carotene supplements will help protect them from cancer, but it can increase the risk of cancer in some populations. Even when a supplement contains what it says, that doesn't mean it's beneficial. Is vitamin C good for you? Yes—if you have scurvy. But for the average person, one of its main effects will be to block some of the positive effects of exercise.

For most people, most of the time, these two conditions don't hold, so supplements are often useless or potentially harmful. Notable exceptions include pregnant women, vegans, people with malabsorption, and many people who are low in vitamin D. In general, though, there's nothing on the market today that meaningfully changes the average person's lifespan. Taking every supplement on the market might lower your bank account, but not your rate of aging.

There's a more seductive kind of supplement that you should be aware of. These aren't basic nutritional supplements, but special supplements formulated around some scientific finding or other. They propose to modulate your biology to make you live longer, but using natural ingredients. Common examples include the antioxidant resveratrol, nicotinamide riboside or the related NMN, and the antioxidant MitoQ. There's nothing wrong with the idea; the only problem is that these supplements mostly don't work, or only help in specific situations. None of them are even close to being as powerful as diet and exercise, which are free and don't have any side effects.

For a healthy dose of skepticism around vitamins and supplements, check out the book *Do You Believe in Magic?* by Paul Offit.

It would be wonderful to be able to buy some extra longevity in a pill but, unless medical tests have identified an acute problem, pills probably only contain false hope. Even if you have identified a problem, unless you're testing again after taking a supplement to see if it fixed the problem, you might still be deluding yourself.

So time spent on supplements should usually be near zero. Most lifestyle optimization time should go to the age-old recommendations: good sleep, sufficient exercise, a healthy diet, mental health, a healthy environment, and full use of modern medicine.

You can get specific recommendations on these things in other longevity books, and there are so many resources out there that it's not worth going into much detail here. Instead, what follows are some general overviews of the topics that you should be aware of and some good books on each one. Remember, these are things that won't work in the long run, but that you should do anyway: sleep, diet, exercise, mental health, vaccines, testing, and health care. If your goal is to be relatively healthy over the course of a normal lifespan, then these lifestyle changes are most of what you need to do. If your goal is to live an unnaturally long lifespan, then lifestyle is merely one small piece of the puzzle.

Sleep is a complex set of processes that keep your body and brain healthy. During sleep, fluids drain out of your brain through the glymphatic system, and this helps flush out molecular waste. Your brain also sends out signals that improve the health of your organs, enhance your immune system, and improve your mental and emotional state. So, sleep has a big influence on how healthy you are and how long you will live. It also helps you make better decisions during the day. If you are sleep deprived you will be less likely to exercise, more likely to eat unhealthy foods, and more likely to end up in stressful situations.

Compared to the average American, optimal sleep could net you a few extra years of life and delay the onset of neurodegenerative diseases by even more than that. Getting optimal sleep can be hard for some people but, for most of us, it's just a matter of developing healthy habits. No eating or screen time right before bed. Reduce blue light exposure at night. A dark, cool bedroom. Maybe read a little before bed and wear socks while you sleep. If you can afford it, buy a sleep tracking device so you can get feedback and improve your sleep routine.

A good resource for how sleep can improve your longevity is *Why We Sleep* by Matthew Walker. It goes into the benefits of sleep, the damage that poor sleep can unleash on your body, and tips for getting the rest that your body needs. It has plenty of motivating studies and practical advice. And you'll finally find out why sleeping from 11 p.m. to 6 a.m. might be better than 1 a.m. to 8 a.m., even though you sleep the same number of hours.

Skipping to the punchline, you should make good sleep a priority in your life rather than something you do begrudgingly at the end of the day. Make it a goal, take it seriously, and put in the effort to make great sleep your status quo. Experiment and figure out how long and what time of night works best for you. Try to discover what rituals or habits will help you get the sleep that will give you the attitude and willpower to live your best life during the day.

Exercise is physical activity that helps maintain your fitness and health. From basics like walking, running, and swimming, to more complex forms of exercise like ice hockey, rock climbing, and weightlifting, exercise strongly shapes how healthy you are and how long you will live. The benefits of exercise come from several avenues. First, damage to your muscles and bones leads to repair, but the repair process can get you to an even stronger state than when you started. This is called hormesis, and the benefits aren't just for your muscles, but also for your cardiovascular system, metabolism, respiratory system, and brain health.

Second, exercise helps clear waste from tissues by circulating fluids and breaking down buildup. Third, exercise causes your muscles and other organs to produce signals that tell your body to be healthier. They make you feel better, too. The effect size of exercise is strong, and many companies would like to replicate it in a prescription medication. If exercise were a pill, everyone would be taking it.

Compared to the average American, you could live several years longer by getting 90 minutes of exercise each day. This may seem like a difficult amount of exercise to achieve until you realize that you can do whatever kind of exercise you enjoy. Yoga, cycling, swimming, fencing—anything you like. Each of these will give you improved bone density, muscle mass and strength, insulin sensitivity, and reduced inflammation. The biggest benefit comes from changing from no exercise to moderate exercise like walking for an hour. You can get some nice additional benefits if you push yourself a little further, getting your heart rate up, getting out of breath, and generally seeing where your limits are. This doesn't have to be Olympic-level training. You can just run for four minutes, walk for four minutes, and repeat four times.

There are many good books on exercise. For an overview of the benefits of exercise and how to think about it for yourself, check out *Exercised* by Daniel Lieberman. However, the best book for you will be whichever one motivates you to exercise more. So feel free to pick up some others that will get you excited enough to play soccer, surf, or whatever. Videos can also be very educational for proper exercise form and ideas for staying active.

Skipping to the punchline: exercise for 90 minutes a day, trying to get a mix of aerobic and resistance exercise. For example, ride a bike for an hour and then cool off with a swim. Or do a yoga class and follow it up with some weight training. Muscle looks nice, helps protect you from injury, improves your metabolism, and also helps keep your organs healthy through intracellular signaling. If you're older, you may want to focus on building up core strength and leg muscle; this will help offset the risks associated with ever-decreasing muscle mass and tone that come with advanced age.

Diet has a major impact on your health and lifespan. Compared to a standard American diet, a healthy diet could add years to your life. And the best part is, your diet is totally under your control. It's a longevity tactic that's available to everyone today and can even save you money.

Some of the best resources for a longevity-promoting diet are produced by Dr. Michael Greger. His website is nutritionfacts.org and he has a few books. You can start with *How Not to Age*, which examines how the way you eat can help you avoid diseases and live longer. The recommendations are simple, but not easy. Just like an insolent child being told to eat their vegetables, you won't magically start eating more healthily just because someone tells you to. But if you take the time to read his books, with their relentless examples from study after study showing how simple dietary changes can promote health, it will help you transition to a healthier diet. And it's not all or nothing. Even if you can't make it all the way to a perfect diet, just moving in the right direction and picking up some healthy habits will reduce disease and extend your lifespan.

Skipping to the punchline: eat a whole-food, plant-based diet. That means vegetables, beans, whole grains, fruits, nuts, and spices. Dr. Greger goes to extreme lengths to make it easier to transition to a whole-food, plant-based diet by providing motivation, recipes, and humor.

If you're on a standard American diet, you will have a difficult time adjusting. The difficulty isn't in the taste of the food. All of these foods are delicious and can be prepared in amazing ways. The difficulty is convenience. Eating what you're used to, what you grew up with, and what is available at restaurants, is easy. Cooking the meals that you're familiar with is easy. Avoiding animal products and unhealthy vegan foods like cookies and potato chips is hard, especially at a barbecue or your best friend's birthday party. Or maybe you've had a hard day at work. Or maybe you've never cooked whole-food plant-based recipes before.

There are a million excuses why you can't eat healthily right now. However, if you want to live as long as possible, you are what is known as a vitalist. A vitalist eating the standard American diet is like a doctor smoking. It goes against what you stand for and, if you want to maximize your survival chances, you'll need to put in the effort to adjust your diet.

You don't have to pay for fancy meal delivery services, pre-packaged foods, or special shakes. You don't need to go on crazy diets where you only eat steak topped with sour cream. Just start making a whole-food, plant-based diet your default, and move as far in that direction as you can. Oatmeal with berries for breakfast, lentil and barley soup for lunch, and maybe some roasted bell peppers, onions, carrots, and fava beans for dinner. Frozen bananas with crushed nuts for dessert. These are all flavorful options that will save you money, keep you trim and healthy, and help you live longer.

Note that a whole-food, plant-based diet isn't the same as a vegan diet. You can have a diet that's both totally vegan and totally unhealthy. Potato chips, cookies, vegan ice cream, and many hyperprocessed foods are all vegan, but they aren't good for you. Just think of juicing machines that take an apple, remove the healthy fiber and vitamin-rich skin, and just give you the water and sugar. Not good. But don't focus on avoiding these unhealthy foods. Instead, try to stuff yourself with healthy foods so you're never tempted by unhealthy ones in the first place.

Eating healthy food gives your body the building blocks it needs to keep all your various metabolic pathways running smoothly. It challenges your body with mildly toxic natural molecules that make you stronger. It helps you maintain a healthy microbiome that then works for your benefit in a variety of ways. It also helps avoid the damaging influence of excess fat on the body. Too much fat puts you at risk of injury, contributes to metabolic disease, and sends detrimental signals throughout your body, causing problems like inflammation.

One last takeaway is that you don't need to dramatically reduce your eating to lose weight; you just need to eat the amount that would maintain the body weight you want to achieve. Picture yourself at your ideal weight, think about how much food you would need to stay at that weight, and start eating that much now. Your body will then naturally shift to your ideal body weight without any harsh dieting.

Mental health has a big influence on your longevity. You might even say mental state has the biggest impact, because it influences all the other factors. To be fair, sleep, exercise, and diet also affect mental state. Still, you can improve it in many ways beyond those areas: socializing, playing games, reading, art, and more. You should also avoid common stressors such as unhealthy relationships and doomscrolling.

Compared with a typical mix of mental and emotional stressors, a healthy attitude and positive environment can add a few years to your life. Factors such as low stress levels, strong social relationships, love, and support are associated with reduced risks of chronic diseases and lower mortality rates. You may have heard that stress can kill you; it's not just a story. Bereavement, depression, and despair all take a measurable toll, and chronic stress contributes to cardiovascular disease and weakens the immune system. In one large cohort study, people who reported a lot of stress and believed it was harming their health had about a 40% higher risk of premature death than people with low stress.

If you have opportunities for mental or emotional improvement, spend some time researching ways to resolve or ease them. Get help if you need it. Living with stress, depression, or other problems lowers not only the quality of your life but the length of it as well.

It's not all downside risk, though. There are many things you can do to improve your mental and emotional health and improve your odds of living longer. The goal is to learn healthy habits for optimizing your own mental and emotional well-being. This includes looking internally at things you can work on, as well as finding external changes you can make to create a supportive and healthy environment. Fostering positive emotions like happiness, gratitude, optimism, and life satisfaction is associated with lower mortality rates. How you do that is up to you, but taking "me time" can help you think proactively about what will make a difference for you. Maybe try painting, cold plunges, karaoke, or whatever. Other things that are commonly helpful are mindfulness practices, giving thanks, meditation, nature walks, and doing things for others. Physical activity can also boost your mood and reduce stress hormones.

Surrounding yourself with things and people that make you happy is also important. Social media can be beneficial in some situations, like keeping up with distant friends or relatives, but it isn't a substitute for in-person interactions. Too much social media can lead to feelings of loneliness and depression. So join a book club, a bike club, a volleyball club, or a bridge club, but somehow get out into the real world and give your body and mind the stimulation they need to thrive.

Meeting people in the real world also helps you form stronger bonds. The stronger your relationship, the more emotional support you will have when you need it, and the greater sense of purpose you will have as you go through life. So don't just look at posts, but give someone a call. Or better yet, invite them out for tea, or a walk in some natural environment. If you're skeptical of the idea that socializing has a big impact on longevity, consider this. Studies have found that the supportive relationship people form with the staff running clinical trials can be a powerful driver of how well they do, sometimes rivaling the effect of the treatment being tested—a sign that human connection itself can have real therapeutic power.

Also, please don't discount the value of professional support. It's cheaper and easier than ever to get therapy, counseling, or to join support groups thanks to video conferencing and online tools. Sharing experiences and challenges with others can help achieve a better mental state. This is true even if you aren't dealing with the "serious issues" that are traditionally associated with professional help. Just as you can hire a physical trainer to support your efforts to improve your physique, you can hire a therapist to train your mental and emotional strength. This is true even if you don't feel you need help or expect therapy to help.

So, optimizing mental and emotional health by reducing stress, fostering strong relationships, and cultivating positive emotions can significantly increase life expectancy. Moreover, it will make you happier.

A useful book on this topic is *Resilient* by Rick Hanson. To skip to the punchline, developing a set of skills around mental wellness requires effort in the beginning, but can lead to habits that make you stronger in the long run. You don't need to do everything that might help, only what works for you, be it meditation, journaling, or building and maintaining supportive relationships.

Another lifestyle choice is where you decide to live. Your environment can have a big impact on your health. One of the most well-studied factors is air pollution. If you live somewhere with poor air quality, it can increase your risk for many diseases, including cardiovascular disease, cancer, and neurodegeneration. Similarly, noisy places might impact your sleep. Other factors include proximity to friends and family, access to health care, water quality, risk of violent crime, and environmental hazards like insect-borne illnesses and natural disasters like wildfires. Extreme temperatures, poor road safety, and indoor hazards like radon, lead, and mold can also shorten your life.

Of course, you need to weigh the risks realistically. For most people, junk food is more likely to kill you than a tornado, so don't over-optimize for things just because they sound scary. The point is just to consider how your location can impact your chances of living long enough to live forever. Embrace the benefits and mitigate the risks.

Just bear in mind that a longevity-promoting place typically has clean air and water, abundant green space, safe and walkable neighborhoods, low exposure to environmental toxins, and ready access to high-quality health care. By contrast, a particularly harmful location might be physically dangerous, have high pollution, or even be near hazardous waste. Even when holding constant things like socioeconomic status, the net difference in life expectancy between the most and least favorable environments within the U.S. can exceed five years.

One final consideration for location is access to longevity technology. If you sign up for cryonics, you will want a living situation that makes it easy for the cryonics company to come and get you, so a cabin in the woods on top of a mountain would not be ideal, no matter how good the air is. You will also want a living situation where people will notice if you kick the bucket. Get a roommate, or at least some nosy neighbors.

This applies to replacement and bioengineering as well. You'll be more likely to find out and take advantage of new therapies as they come out if you're close to where they are available. The key metric here isn't physical distance, but how easy it is to get there. So living near an airport or other transportation hub could be useful.

While radical life extension will require new technologies, existing technologies can help you right now. These include vaccines, testing, and health care. Vaccines carry some risk, so you shouldn't necessarily hunt down every vaccine on the planet. With that said, you wouldn't want to die from some disease that could have been prevented or at least mitigated with a simple injection. So take all the common vaccines for your area and get special vaccines if you're traveling so you're covered in the area you're going to. Vaccines have some risk, but the risk of dying from the diseases vaccines prevent is far higher than the risk from the vaccine.

Testing is also very valuable. Testing means taking measurements of some of your biomarkers, which indicate how healthy you are. For example, common biomarkers include your weight, blood cholesterol levels, and your blood pressure. Many different biomarkers exist, with many ways to measure them. Traditional types of testing require occasionally getting a blood panel, urine analysis, poop tests, and skin screens. These give very useful information, but are hard to perform and can be costly. Newer tests are becoming available that allow for cheap testing at home through mail-in kits.

Testing is not only getting cheaper and easier, but new tests are being developed that can help you track your health and detect problems early. Blood tests in development can detect cancer, neurodegenerative diseases, and more. With a large budget, you could take hundreds of tests every month to keep a close eye on your health. There are even expensive clinics that will help you do just that. Clinics also have large testing equipment that can scan your body and generate more holistic data.

Not only are more tests available every year, but the pace of testing is speeding up with wearables. You can purchase wearable electronics that give real-time information about a limited set of biomarkers. A popular example is a continuous glucose monitor that sticks to your upper arm and reports blood sugar levels to your phone. This can help you see how your body responds to different foods and eating schedules. There are also electronic rings and bracelets that can track your heart rate, sleep quality, and so on. These aren't just for fun, they can tell you when something is wrong. Researchers are developing apps that can tell you when you're sick before you get symptoms, just by looking at wearable data. Getting help before you're really sick could save your life.

Another particularly useful test is gene sequencing. As we learn more about how gene variants affect longevity, you'll want to know if you're at risk for heart disease, cancer, and neurodegeneration, so you can take preventative measures as early as possible. Knowing your genome will also help you take advantage of gene editing therapies as they become available.

On top of gene sequencing, you can also have your epigenome tested. Your epigenome can give you a rough sense of how biologically old you are, as opposed to your chronological age. These aging clocks don't yet give specific recommendations on how to improve your health, but they can give you a general sense of how you're doing.

So depending on your circumstances, do your annual blood tests with your doctor or take advantage of other newer tests that are coming out that can give you more information. If you can afford it, consider going to a clinic that runs hundreds of tests over two days. If not, find the tests that are most relevant to your personal and family history and start with those. Knowing that something is wrong early can make it much easier to treat, and treating something early can add years to your life.

Testing is also important because human biology is highly variable, so advice that's good for most people might be bad for you. For example, even broccoli, the thing everyone agrees is good for you, isn't good for you if you're allergic to it, or if you have certain thyroid conditions, low iodine, or specific gastrointestinal conditions. The best way to know what works for you is to test yourself, understand your baseline biomarkers, and then see how different lifestyle changes impact them. This is true for each and every topic: sleep, exercise, diet, and so on.

Run tests on yourself, track your biomarkers, go see your doctor, and take medications if you need them. Do whatever you can to increase your chances of staying alive until there's a radical shift in longevity technology.

Normal health care is also valuable. If you have a suspicion that something is wrong, go see a doctor. Many people die every year because they ignore obvious signs and symptoms of serious conditions like heart attack, stroke, pneumonia, and so on. Antibiotics can save your life, but only if you take them before you get sepsis. Similarly, clot-busting drugs can save you after a heart attack or stroke, but only in the first few hours. So make sure you have a doctor and know where to go for urgent and emergency care.

Key Takeaways

Healthy choices may be guaranteed to fail, but they are also very likely to help. Lifestyle can affect the accumulation rate of both intrinsically repairable and irreparable damage. If you're young, you might not need to worry about certain types of damage because your body is still stable and can withstand those kinds of factors. Being out in extreme heat might be uncomfortable, but will be much less life-threatening for a younger adult than for someone of advanced age. The older you get, the more careful you should be with your lifestyle.

Regardless of individual circumstances, everyone can use healthy choices and a longevity-focused lifestyle to live longer and more happily, and to be more effective in the pursuit of radical life extension. So learn about the impact of sleep, exercise, diet, and more, so you can make the most of them.

Finally, consider the most important lifestyle choice of all. That means choosing how much of your life and resources to dedicate to the technology needed for radical life extension. In the end, biostasis, replacement, and advanced bioengineering are the only things that can save the lives of the people you care about. As much as possible, buttress your life with these technologies and healthy habits to gain extra months, years, and, perhaps, decades.

There's no telling what might happen and there are many ways for the future to unfold. As you imagine how things may play out, remember that your choices can influence which predictions come true. The right decision, however small, could make the difference between a normal life and an extraordinary one.

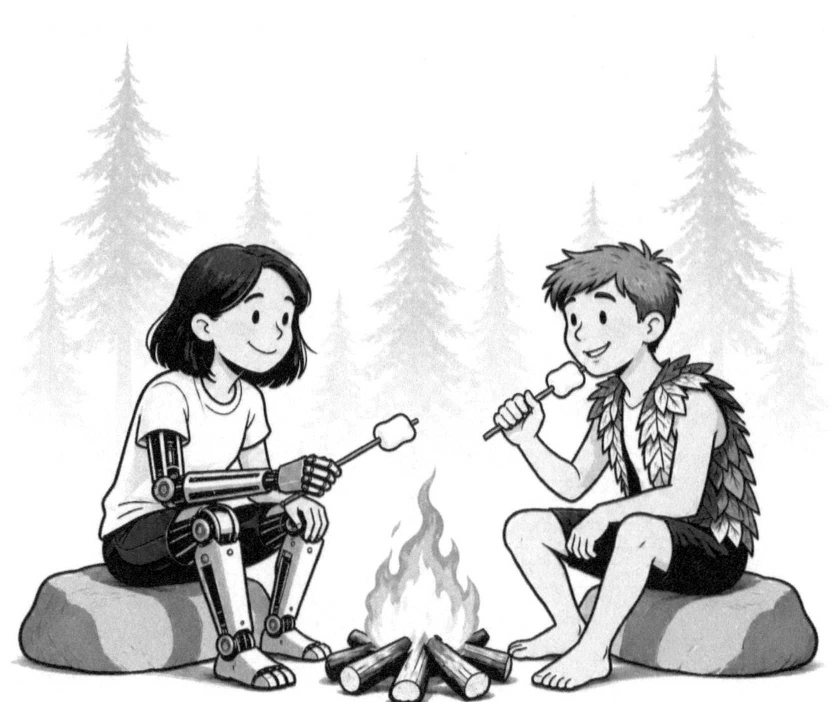

CHAPTER 10

SPECULATIONS

The future is uncertain, but it's worth imagining how the pieces might actually fit together. Following are a few ways the road to radical life extension could unfold.

These are conjectures about what may lead to indefinite lifespan. They don't represent what will happen, but what could happen. What actually happens depends on you, so visualize success and then make it happen.

A Biostasis Timeline

For many years, biostasis continues to be the only option for people who don't want to die, but it remains a small community. Membership grows slowly from the thousands to tens of thousands, and eventually the service is available almost everywhere.

Scientists continue to doggedly push the boundaries of what is possible, developing new cryoprotectants and rewarming technology. Then there's a small breakthrough. A rat is vitrified and rewarmed successfully. Not just one rat, but three out of 100 that were tested are revived and retain their memories of a maze that they were trained on.

Cryonics memberships grow, but even greater is the rate at which people choose to preserve their pets. People seem to think that if it works for a rat, maybe the process can save their childhood cat or dog as well. As pet longevity seeps through culture, human longevity sees a corresponding increase in popularity.

Shortly after that, human kidneys are shown to survive vitrification, which begins to ease the organ shortage. Hearts become the second organ cryopreserved and then successfully transplanted. Organ banking becomes a going concern, and people begin to wait not just for an organ, but an organ particularly well-suited to their needs.

Then the first nonhuman primate is successfully vitrified and revived. The monkey's memory seems to be largely intact, recognizing caretakers, toys, and playmates. Shortly thereafter cryonics becomes generally accepted as plausible. Some hospitals and hospices switch from tolerating the practice to offering it as a standard option for disposition of remains. Soon everyone knows someone who is waiting in biostasis.

As it becomes more popular, the cost of biostasis drops steadily. It moves from an option that requires large savings or advanced planning to something the average person can afford when they are making last-minute end-of-life plans.

Then the stars align. A 25-year-old woman is diagnosed with untreatable breast cancer. She chooses to go into biostasis, and is preserved with a new generation of technologies that prevent both ice formation and cracking, all without toxicity. Just seven years later, her cancer becomes completely curable via engineered immune cells. Five years after that, experiments in pigs demonstrate that the latest rewarming technology is ready to revive anyone cryopreserved with the latest generation of cryoprotectants. Before rewarming the young woman, they take a small sample of her skin cells and convert them into cancer-fighting immune cells. With the cure in hand, they revive her and give her the good news: she is cancer free.

Many people remain in biostasis long after that, having been preserved with older technologies. Newer techniques are developed to repair ice damage and more people are revived. Technology to repair cracks is invented and even more people come out of biostasis. At the same time, people continue to enter biostasis for a variety of reasons: accidents, incurable diseases, and the like. But their stays are typically much shorter than the original cryonauts who entered biostasis in the latter half of the 20th century.

Biostasis becomes a normal part of health care. Many prefer to go to a hospital that has staff and equipment on hand to cryopreserve patients who are terminally ill or injured. Not everyone chooses biostasis, but almost everyone at least has the option.

A Biostasis Scenario

Your own circumstances also shape your strategy.

First, suppose you're 90. Maybe you have no savings, no family, and no friends. Your family died in a freak accident. You attended the funeral of each of your friends, whom you outlived mainly through luck. Whether it was good luck or bad luck seems unclear at times.

You're a magnet for ill fortune, or so your doctor tells you at your regular checkup. You can't afford a good doctor, and the one you do have has a terrible bedside manner. With a disinterested yawn, he reveals to you that you have several incurable cancers and he estimates you have a few months to live. On the bright side, your brain is fine, so you will get to fully experience your rapid decline and lonely end.

No replacement or bioengineering solutions will come fast enough to save you. Your only option is biostasis, but you can't get an insurance contract to cover the cost of cryonics. Walking home, you make a decision—you decide not to give up.

You post a crowdfunding campaign online to raise money for your own chemopreservation, but you only get a tiny donation and even that seems like an accident. You abandon that strategy and look for jobs that you can start quickly. You find two and work like mad for your remaining months, making just enough money to pay for the relatively inexpensive chemopreservation. Since you have a terminal diagnosis, it's easy to get approval for medical aid in dying, which allows you to schedule your procedure ahead of time and get the laboratory-grade preservation quality.

Forty years after that, you're moved from your original refrigerator to a larger facility. Just after the one-hundredth anniversary of your preservation, the first chemopreserved patient is revived. Biostasis is a first-in-last-out game, so it's another 60 years before you're revived. While you look 25 years old in your new body, you briefly hold the title of oldest living person.

There are still many more waiting in biostasis, so it becomes your turn to help those who came before.

A Biostasis and Bioengineering Scenario

Now, suppose instead you're in a better situation. You have always taken good care of yourself. You look younger than your age, and younger than your friends. But as you turn 45, you start to feel older, and by 60 you're looking a little older than you would like. Fortunately, longevity therapies start to hit the market. You take advantage of all of them and, along with a fairly healthy lifestyle, you continue to age better than your peers. While you're still doing pushups in your 80s, many of your friends are pushing up daisies. Gene therapies keep your cardiovascular system unnaturally healthy. They also keep your muscles lean and your skin tight. There's no solution for everything, but you buy extra years with yearly injections and continue working long past retirement age to save a longevity nest egg.

Things start to go downhill around your 107th birthday. Your brain is much healthier than those few of your generation who are still around after over a century of normal aging, and you're relatively sharp. However, you're starting to have trouble remembering things. You find a new doctor after outliving your previous one. Your new doctor tells you that you have done everything right. Thanks to your lifestyle and adoption of new longevity technology, you have lived a few decades longer and are in much better shape than you would have been otherwise. Still, he says, time is catching up with you and you're likely to develop neurodegenerative disease within the next five years.

You decide to go into biostasis before your brain has time to deteriorate, giving yourself a three-year target. You invest a large fraction of your savings into research and development of gene therapies that could improve the cryopreservation process. Four years later there has been a lot of technological progress but also some cognitive decline. You decide the time has come.

You pack up some memorabilia, have a goodbye party, and travel to a cryonics facility. After two weeks of preparations, including two gene therapies that you funded, you go into cryostasis. Though you still end up in the dewar, the additional time and effort gain you the use of the latest technology and lead to a spectacular preservation quality.

You spend only 27 years in biostasis. When you come out, almost everyone you know is still alive thanks to the continued progress of longevity and biostasis technology, including your own contributions.

A Replacement Timeline

Consider a timeline where people reach indefinite lifespan solely through replacement technologies.

In the near term, fluid replacement therapies are developed that build on therapeutic plasma exchange. They reduce chronic inflammation as well as the accumulation of extracellular debris. Techniques are developed for restoring drainage of cerebrospinal fluid, such as shunts. These prevent the toxic buildup of protein aggregates in the brain and delay neurodegenerative disease.

Around the same time, mitochondrial transplantation becomes commonplace. These therapies deliver young, healthy mitochondria systemically, which enhances cell and tissue function throughout the body. People begin to have the energy to exercise, continue working, and maintain a healthy lifestyle for much longer than before.

Shortly thereafter, ECM particle injections are developed that allow the extracellular matrix of tissues and organs to be rejuvenated. The first ones target the skin because it's easy to access. However, once people see their skin getting younger, the same techniques are applied to internal organs. Younger ECM helps muscles maintain lean mass, prevents fibrosis and undesirable shifts in cell populations in various organs, and improves tissue function wherever the particles can be safely injected.

Then the next generation of cell therapies enters the clinic. These have improved cell characteristics and better delivery methods. Some bolster the immune system against specific diseases, but others provide a way to reduce chronic inflammation and restore youthful levels of various cell populations.

Some cell replacement therapies are so effective that organs are able to maintain youthful function. In particular, various cell populations in the brain are kept young and healthy, allowing better support and health of neurons. This helps maintain brain connectivity and reduce the loss of brain volume over time.

In some organs, cell replacement alone doesn't work, but cells and ECM in combination provide benefits. Some tissues and organs can be kept in a state of greatly extended health with infusions of young ECM and young cells. Large quantities of cell transplants also lead to reduced risk of cancer, as transplanted cells don't have a lifetime of accumulated DNA damage.

Human cells aren't the only things that begin to be replaced regularly. Young, healthy combinations of gut microbiota are given to patients periodically, helping to support the gut as well as immune function and brain health. Optimized combinations of youthful microbiota are developed for every part of the body, for instance in the mouth and on the skin. Rather than trying to disinfect everything, people simply crowd-out bad bacteria with ones that are beneficial.

But with all of this progress, aging marches on. People are healthier and live longer on average, but not enough to reach longevity escape velocity.

Then the organ shortage is solved and everything changes.

Tissues and organs become available for anyone who might want one. Skin transplants not only make people look younger, but actually improve the protective barrier around the body against injury and infection.

Many over the age of 50 begin to get a second thymus, implanted into their lower abdomen. Similarly, some begin to proactively get a third kidney before their original kidneys begin to fail. Eventually, leg transplantation becomes a safe and effective way to improve mobility, metabolic health, and immune function.

Immune rejection is solved and people no longer need genetically identical replacement parts. Everyone gets the best version of every cell, tissue, and organ.

As robotic surgical platforms improve, people begin to opt for multivisceral transplants, getting young versions of half or all of their internal organs. Neurodegenerative disease declines as improved support from young kidneys, the liver, and the immune system improves brain health. Some artificial organs begin to surpass their biological equivalents. The elderly with artificial lenses can see twice as well as normal young adults. People can begin to depend on artificial hearts to keep them alive for decades.

Eventually, human tissue constructs are developed that contain everything except the brain, allowing for body transplants below the neck. People can have their old and busted bodies removed and replaced with young, healthy ones. Along with the body, the face, eyes, scalp, and ears are transplanted so the patient looks young all over. The recovery period lasts months, but afterwards patients are back out in the world. More importantly, their chance of developing age-related diseases is reset to youthful levels.

With a young body, the brain lasts much longer, but it still ages. Cell transplants help keep brain cell populations young and healthy. ECM transplants in the prefrontal cortex, hippocampus, amygdala, and temporal association cortices help keep those systems youthful. Tissue transplantation of the cerebellum, brainstem, and primary motor and sensory areas allows them to be kept healthy as well.

While the first round of replacement is patchy and piecemeal, these early technologies allow people to live additional decades on average. Over those decades, the technology improves to the point where replacement is standardized, safe, and effective. People begin to get annual infusions of cells and ECM along with their yearly checkup. Each transplant not only makes them younger but also improves their health to the best possible level with current technology. When necessary, automated robotic surgeries provide completely new kidneys, lungs, or other body parts.

Aging is never stopped. Cells continue to accumulate damage. Fluids and ECM also continue to degrade. Yet eventually, thanks to replacement, aging no longer matters. External supplies of young cells, fluids, and tissues lead to the continual renewal of the human body and an indefinite lifespan.

A Replacement Scenario

Suppose you live near a wooded mountain. You spend your evenings hiking through pine forests and watching plants and animals try to survive in the brutal reality of nature.

In your 40s, you notice that you're having trouble seeing the details of flowers that you pass along the trail. Then you get some artificial lenses and can see better than ever. Five years later, you notice that you can't quite hike as long or as high as you used to. Then you start getting annual mitochondria infusions and your muscles seem to vibrate with youthful vigor.

In your 50s, as you hike along a favorite route, you stop to look at your reflection in a secluded mountain lake. To your despair, your skin is starting to look thin and saggy. You call your longevity clinic, and they bring you in for a four-day skin overhaul, with injections of ECM particles covered in cells. For a few days, you look like you ran naked through a cactus patch. After you recover, you notice your skin looks and feels younger, and the occasional scratch in the woods heals much more quickly.

Five years later, you decide to be a little proactive and purchase microbiome replacement products. The best bacteria from around the world are mailed to you in the forms of toothpaste, skin cream, and food, among others. At your next checkup, your doctor notes improvements to cognitive function, immune function, and other biomarkers.

In your 60s you notice that you're having trouble hearing some of the bird songs you always love listening to in the summer. Then you get a hearing aid and it's no trouble at all. Five years later, your doctor says it may be time to consider some more advanced procedures.

All the hiking has taken a toll on your knees and ankles, so you're tempted to buy a new pair of legs. However, you decide to dip your toe into the water first and get a new thymus. The surgery is quick and easy, and you go home the same day. A few years later, you decide to go big and replace all of your internal organs. It's a serious surgery, but the robots are fast and efficient. After some bed rest, you can hardly believe how much easier it is to breathe.

About a decade later you reach your original life expectancy. With all of the replacement therapies you have taken advantage of, you're biologically half your age, and your doctor expects you will live another 30 years. However, the Grim Reaper gets impatient and sends a bear after you. You get mauled badly, but are found and brought to the emergency room.

You wake up a few months later. Your doctor explains that they couldn't repair your injuries, so they performed a body transplant. Now instead of 30 years, he expects you will live four decades. A hooded figure outside your window shakes his bony fist.

Over the next four decades your annual replacement therapies focus more and more on brain health and your doctor gives up on guessing how long you will live.

A Biostasis and Replacement Scenario

Suppose you have an older friend who is on death's door. He signs up for brain-only biostasis and one day gets vitrified and put into a dewar.

The facility happens to be near a place you like to go for vacation, so every year you make a habit of stopping by to check up on him. Over time, more and more people are stored in the facility. You get to know many of their friends and relatives. Year after year, you all come back to visit and share stories. That's until reversal of cryopreservation seems to start working.

Suddenly, everyone is in a hurry to get their people out of biostasis. Someone who died of a heart attack is warmed up and given a new heart. Someone who died of respiratory disease is given new lungs. Your friend needs more than an organ or two, though. He needs a whole new body.

No problem, says the staff. Bodyoids have been available for many years. They order one and make some bone marrow from cells in your friend's skull, which is then transplanted into the bodyoid to prevent immune rejection. They move your friend into a medical pod that clears out his vasculature, adds cells and ECM where needed, and performs other repairs. Repairs continue as he is warmed up, right up until the moment he is placed into the bodyoid. You think he looks different from before, but it has been so long that you can't quite remember.

While looking through old photos to refresh your memory, you try to decide what you should do to celebrate.

A Bioengineering Timeline

Consider another timeline where people reach an indefinite lifespan solely through bioengineering technologies. The main technologies here are gene therapies, delivered directly into the body or to cells that are then transfused back into the body.

Over the next decade, several helpful gene therapies become available. They don't cure aging, but they alleviate many of the common age-related changes in metabolism and reduce many of the common causes of death. And they make you look great, too.

Fat is a major target of early gene therapies and, after some treatments, your body no longer accumulates excess fat. Subcutaneous fat is kept at a healthy minimum, with a favorable mix of brown fat. Fat infiltration of organs is prevented. Muscles and bones are made strong and resistant to atrophy. Falling simultaneously becomes less dangerous and less common.

Similarly, bioengineering technology brings cholesterol levels under control. Excess free cholesterol and oxidized cholesterol are things of the past, greatly reducing the incidence of stroke and heart attack. Not only that, but improved cardiovascular health and blood flow improve the function of your brain and other organs.

Better control of cell populations is achieved, first with powerful senolytics that are developed to periodically destroy lingering senescent cells. Removing these cells cuts down on inflammation and reduces cancer risk. Similarly, powerful antibacterial peptide production is installed in your genome, allowing your body to more effectively fight off pathogens. Meanwhile, super microbiota are developed that not only produce more helpful metabolites but also outcompete harmful species. This takes your gut health above what is expected for a healthy individual your age and, in many ways, above that of a young person. Super-healthy guts lead to improvements in immune function, cardiovascular health, and brain health.

Even certain types of cancer become curable through gene therapies. The treatments produce CAR-T cells in vivo, and alter immune cells to make them resistant to confusing signals from the tumor microenvironment, among other strategies.

Improvements are also made in waste clearance. New enzymes become available that can break down most intracellular and extracellular aggregates. Lipofuscin is no longer an issue. AGE-breaking enzymes clear cross-links from the extracellular matrix, restoring not only tissue elasticity and function, but also healthy cell behavior as cells begin to receive youthful signals from the rejuvenated ECM.

Similarly, misfolded proteins begin to be cleared from both inside cells and the extracellular matrix. The heart no longer suffers from the buildup of transthyretin, and the body is given genes to produce enzymes that break up other types of protein aggregates. Prions are wiped out with the same strategy.

Additional ECM repair is done through specially modified cells. For example, some cells are programmed to produce young elastin precursors and to lay them down effectively in various tissues. Other cells are developed that can detect damaged ECM and remodel it, improving health in all tissues, but especially in the vasculature.

Speaking of the vasculature, gene and cell therapies are developed to maintain youthful levels of capillary density in all tissues. The improved blood flow helps support tissue function, especially in the muscles and brain. Older, stiff vasculature is slowly degraded and replaced with newly grown arteries and veins.

Yet, the two primary obstacles to radical life extension continue to stand like immovable statues: the delivery problem and the design problem.

And then, one day, there is a breakthrough—a team of engineers finds a way to deliver gene therapies safely and reliably to every cell. Any changes that can help in any way are now available. Patients can get their preferred version of each gene, changing not only their eye and hair color, but also their probability of developing aging pathology. DNA repair is strengthened with genetic machinery from other species as well as artificial genes produced by engineers. In addition, RNA and protein production are improved with new transcription and translation machinery.

Mitochondrial DNA is moved into the nucleus, keeping both mitochondria and energy-hungry tissues like skeletal muscle and the brain healthy. Antiviral machinery is installed in all cells. Chronic infections are systematically wiped out. All transposable elements are disabled.

Even as cancer becomes rarer, it becomes more easily detectable at the earliest stages. Custom treatments can be produced quickly, and long-term survival rates are high.

Later, tissue regeneration is enabled for adult humans. Tiny amounts of tissue can be removed throughout any organ, allowing it to regrow healthy tissue in place. It becomes possible to program cells to degrade old ECM safely, allowing young, healthy ECM to be laid down in its place. Many tissues and organs can be rebuilt in place, without disrupting their function.

Many diseases are cured, others are mitigated, but aging rages on. The design problem turns out to be harder than anyone expected. Too big a knot for any person to untangle. So enormous data sets are collected to characterize both genes and gene networks. Along with unprecedented levels of computational power, this unlocks AI tools that help bioengineers design solutions to problems that were previously insurmountable.

Bioengineering reaches a technological level where, while not all damage can be prevented, all major types of damage can be repaired. Age-related disease continues to evolve as people start to live long enough for previously unimportant types of damage to accumulate to pathological levels. Yet new solutions continue to emerge at faster and faster rates and the human genome is continually improved. While a perfect solution is not yet available, aging is no longer a major driver of mortality, and accounts for fewer and fewer deaths each year.

A Bioengineering Scenario

Suppose that you're born at just the right time, which unfortunately means everyone older than you was born too early. Real longevity technologies emerge in your 30s, and you benefit from them. They make you healthier throughout your life, and your life expectancy, while not indefinite, rises quickly. You're wealthy enough to afford even the most advanced therapies. As a result, you get a few decades older but your life expectancy jumps by decades as well.

Not everything is perfect, though. The annual injections you get keep most of your body in good shape, but some parts continue to age. When you reach your 80s, you begin to wonder if science and technology will be able to save you. Just as your kidney function starts to look a little shaky, you see an ad for a new gene therapy that takes care of it.

Time marches on, but so does progress in bioengineering. Each year a new scheme for slowing aging is devised. Just as frequently new ideas emerge for repairing age-related damage. Every time you worry you're running out of time, someone winds your clock a little.

Still, it's a near thing. You go through the aging process and suffer the agonies of old age. Chronic diseases pile up, albeit slowly. Eventually the pendulum shifts and, after you turn 100, every birthday brings you closer to being young again.

A Replacement and Bioengineering Timeline

Consider another potential timeline in which replacement and bioengineering work together to create the shortest path to radical life extension.

Replacement therapies for mitochondria and microbiota are small early hits. Gene therapies take cardiovascular disease and cancer down a notch.

Amid a variety of minor new therapies, bioengineering lands a huge breakthrough by solving the hardest problem in replacement: supply. Human cells are edited so that they will grow into tissue constructs that can then be used for any replacement therapy. The organ shortage is solved, and young, immune-matched cells of every type are suddenly available.

The transplant industry begins to grow rapidly, treating all incurable diseases with young, disease-free tissues and organs. The benefits of young tissue and organs are evident, as the incidence of age-related disease declines with the amount of tissue replaced. It's suddenly safer to be a 70-year-old with 20-year-old organs than a 50-year-old with their original organs.

Replacement creates a fast track for gene therapies to be transferred into the body because all the new cells, tissues, and organs being transplanted into patients have genetic enhancements. They not only have the benefit of being younger, but they also stay younger longer and perform better than natural young cells and organs. Every gene therapy can enter the replacement supply chain and bypass the problem of direct delivery completely.

Shortly thereafter, the problem of immune rejection is solved. The replacement industry grows even faster now that generic, off-the-shelf cells, tissues, and organs can be made at scale. The cost of replacement therapies begins to decrease quickly, even while the benefits continue to increase.

Not all organs and tissues are easily replaceable, but bioengineering comes through with a solution to the engraftment problem. Suddenly, cells can be administered that will take up residence in existing tissue and replace their older, less functional predecessors. Cells in tissues can be replaced gradually rather than through surgery. This doesn't solve every problem, but young cells greatly reduce the incidence of cancer and other diseases.

It also buys time for bioengineering therapies to be developed that can solve some of the harder problems, especially the rejuvenation of the brain.

At this point, the brain remains the most challenging and most important problem in radical life extension. All the power of bioengineering and replacement converges on the seat of consciousness, and solutions are found. Gene therapies are produced that regrow the vasculature in place. Specialized cells are designed that can home in on specific regions of the brain and turn over the ECM. Replacement cells can be injected to swap out the entire glial population. A new type of cell is created that can engage neurons to exchange their nuclei for fresh copies. Gene therapies allow neurons to clear intracellular junk. Some neurons are just swapped wholesale.

Before we know it, aging is under control. Not completely solved, but in a place where people start to wonder if death really gives meaning to life, or if we just said that to make ourselves feel better.

Key Takeaways

Having looked at a few scenarios, it should be clear that there are many paths to victory. What's more, we can get to radical life extension without relying on a long-shot scientific breakthrough or some other miracle. The most practical approach is to shift resources into effective strategies and put in the work to make the new technologies we require.

We don't know exactly how the future will play out. We don't know exactly which technological roadmap will get us there. But we do know the direction that we need to move in, and the first steps to take in that direction. We also know that how quickly these kinds of scenarios play out depends on how much work goes into making them happen. That depends on what you and every other person decide to do with your lives. Fortunately, there are many ways to spend our lives saving lives.

Now it's just a race against the clock.

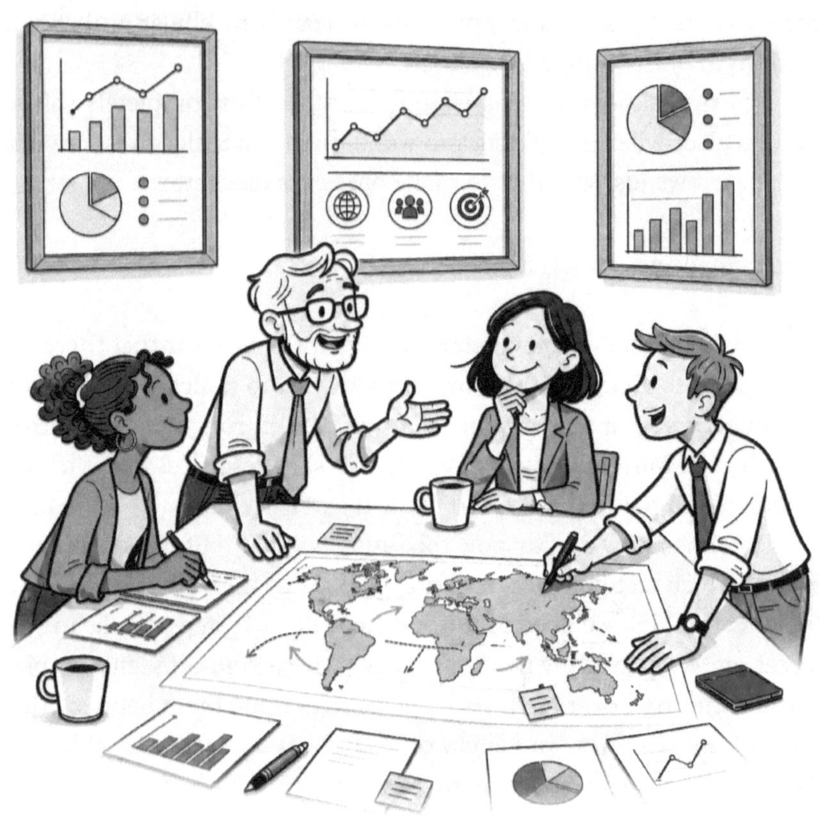

CHAPTER 11

SAVING LIVES

Whether you want to save yourself, your friends and family, or everyone, many things must happen to make that goal a reality. Radical life extension won't emerge from a secret lab run by a small cabal. It will come from the coordinated efforts of thousands of people, each contributing different skills, resources, and ideas. No one can do everything, so for anyone who seriously wants to live forever or die trying, the real question is how to spend your limited time and attention.

If you can only do one thing, make sure the people you care about become biostasis customers. There are multiple providers, so you will need to research which ones operate in your area and offer the services you want.

Arranging biostasis is like committing to a healthy lifestyle. It isn't sufficient on its own, but it's part of any rational plan for radical life extension. Diet and exercise won't get you to longevity escape velocity, and biostasis isn't guaranteed to either. However, biostasis is unique in that it's the only option not guaranteed to fail.

Biostasis matters even if you expect replacement and bioengineering to solve aging soon, because aging is far from the only way you can die. Whether death comes from old age or an accident, a biostasis contract is a life preserver you will want available for everyone you care about.

Once you and your loved ones have biostasis plans in place, you may want to invest some effort in lifestyle optimization. Living conditions and habits that preserve health increase your odds of reaching future therapies. They also improve outcomes if biostasis is needed, since better baseline health enables better preservation.

Most people can do more than push out their preservation date with pushups at the gym. One thing that anybody can do to help is to become a volunteer for cryonics cases. A cryonics case is a team effort, and you don't need to have any special skills. You're trained on how standby, stabilization, and transport work. When a case comes in, you and the rest of the team are dispatched to a patient's location to pick them up and bring them to the long-term care facility. Depending on how you want to be involved, you might assist the team in cooling the patient, administering medications, or just keeping detailed notes. It's not easy work, but it can be rewarding.

Redirecting some effort from personal health toward accelerating longevity technology can also be a good trade-off. If you already exercise an hour a day, adding another hour yields diminishing returns. Spending that time on longevity tech may have a small effect too, but one that applies to everyone: a thousand people exercising more might help a thousand people live a little longer, while a thousand people working on longevity technology could help billions live much longer.

The right balance depends on your situation. If you're sedentary, going from zero to one hour of exercise may buy you years. If you're a scientist working on a genuinely life-extending therapy who commutes on a bicycle, your time may be better spent in the lab. The broader point is that the impact of time and money isn't always obvious, and technological progress is the only path to radical life extension. Everyone who wants to travel that trail should do what they can to blaze it.

Advocacy and Education

If you decide to contribute to technological progress, learn the landscape first: you can help in many ways, but you need context before choosing where to focus.

The fastest way to get up to speed is to connect with the longevity community. Many organizations have people willing to help you get started. Once you're connected, everything moves faster because you gain access to collaborators who want you to succeed. Different groups focus on science, advocacy, investing, or infrastructure. Join the ones most relevant to your goals, and keep networking to find both mentors and people who need your help.

If you're new and want to push hard, consider joining the Longevity Biotech Fellowship. It concentrates scientists, engineers, and investors working on critical-path projects. If your interest is shaping public opinion and building global momentum, join the Vitalism movement, which focuses on mobilizing talent and capital at scale.

The more people who understand the opportunity to radically improve human health, the faster progress will occur. Not everyone will be able to contribute, but some will, and every additional contributor will help more people live long and prosper. Education and outreach are therefore high-impact activities. You don't really understand something until you can teach it, so prove that you've learned something by helping others learn it too.

Many people have strong psychological defenses around death, so it's not just a matter of going door to door. You might start with friends and family, though this can be awkward. In that case, it may be more productive to talk with people who are already curious, or who ask about that cool longevity shirt you're wearing.

Writing articles, essays, or posts can be a way to spread what you learn. You can advocate directly for a world in which death is optional, or start more subtly by focusing on better solutions to age-related disease. For quicker feedback, share infographics, memes, and short content, but never stop dreaming big. Creative projects with wider appeal like art, music, videos, and stories can normalize aging research in ways that technical writing can't. Longer formats like books, documentaries, and journal articles are great to have on hand for people whose curiosity has been piqued and who want to go deeper. Always keep in mind that entertainment and education are better together.

Sometimes it's not what you know, but who you know. If you have access to influencers, encourage them to learn about and promote longevity science. These could be internet personalities, but also leaders in different fields. Teaching scientists, educators, and business leaders can produce network effects within their communities.

Instead of borrowing a community or audience, you could build one yourself. Organizing meetups, conferences, or local groups brings people together and sustains momentum. Volunteering at events is another way to contribute while building relationships. Let everyone know that youth doesn't need to be wasted on the young.

Adjacent fields are also fertile ground. Branching out might not only help you make new connections, but also connect ideas from different industries. Cross-disciplinary collaboration with AI, physics, materials science, and robotics can unlock new approaches to solving aging. Bringing people together for short bursts of work like hackathons, workshops, and special projects can accelerate progress.

You could also build educational platforms, project trackers, or public databases for aging research. And consider your own training. Retraining or working in an aging lab may be a once-in-a-lifetime opportunity, at least until we solve aging.

Longevity technology is being built within a legal and regulatory environment that can either accelerate or strangle progress. Changing that environment is another potential high-impact path. Policymakers respond better when arguments are framed in familiar terms, such as pensions, retirement, health care costs, and economic productivity, so forecasting models of extended lifespan can also help shift attention and funding. Advocacy can also push governments to fund aging research at levels commensurate with its importance. Compared to other programs, aging research remains dramatically underfunded.

Specific legal reforms matter, too. Stronger protections for assisted suicide and explicit inclusion of cryonics in health care directives could improve biostasis outcomes. Faster regulatory pathways and reduced burdens would help replacement and bioengineering therapies reach the clinic sooner. Legal recognition of aging as a treatable condition would significantly strengthen the field.

Patient advocacy can be particularly powerful because regulation cuts both ways. Rules that reduce the risk of unsafe drugs can also delay or block access to therapies that would save lives, and the people lost to those delays make up what some call the invisible graveyard. Reducing unnecessary regulatory friction through grassroots organizing, right-to-try laws that let people access promising drugs years earlier, alternative regulatory frameworks, or even special economic zones can literally save lives, with opportunities at local, regional, and national levels.

Investment and Philanthropy

Philanthropy can have an outsized impact on longevity, especially while the field is still young and many projects struggle to raise capital. You can support existing nonprofits directly, or donate to advocacy organizations that amplify your efforts. If a clear gap exists, creating a new nonprofit may be worthwhile, whether it's focused on scholarships, open-access publishing, journalism, or dedicated research centers.

A more hands-on approach is to identify specific projects to fund, whether they are basic research, data infrastructure, advocacy, or social programs. There are people with the time, energy, and talent to do good work, and they just need financial support to push the field forward.

Then again, you don't need to fund everything yourself. Nonprofits often need help designing programs, writing grants, or aligning longevity goals with their missions. If you can write good proposals, you can unlock funding for important projects.

Prizes for longevity milestones could attract attention and talent in a milestone-driven way. The largest example of this so far is XPRIZE Healthspan, which offered $101 million to teams who find ways to rejuvenate the brain, muscles, and immune system by 20 years. Coordinating high-net-worth individuals or grassroots pledges can mobilize capital that incentivizes progress in important areas, while also building excitement.

Philanthropy can also support human trials, shared standards, or integration of longevity into mainstream medicine. If you talk to someone who cares about effective altruism, consider mentioning that charitable giving toward high-impact longevity work is one of the most effective altruistic actions available.

We're not completely dependent on philanthropy, though. Longevity technology is now mature enough to attract equity investment. If you're finance-minded, you can put your deal-hunting skills to work stalking death. One way is to angel invest directly or through longevity-focused funds. This will not only benefit technological progress, but could give you a financial advantage, because longevity biotech has structural advantages over traditional drug development. Therapies are generally safer, making it more likely that they will pass clinical trials. They will generally help with multiple diseases, giving the companies you invest in many options for commercialization. These therapies also have enormous markets. Tread carefully, though, since most early-stage biotech bets fail.

If you lack the time to research deals, funds or syndicates are viable options. You could also form your own firm, launch an accelerator, or build a venture studio. Public equity products like longevity index funds could bring mainstream capital into the space.

More experimental approaches are possible too. Prediction markets and decentralized science organizations could fund the high-risk rejuvenation programs that traditional investors avoid. Groups like VitaDAO, CryoDAO, and HydraDAO are already deploying crypto funds into very valuable projects.

Alternatively, some people choose to work outside aging to build capital to then bring back into the field. This could certainly help, as funding remains a major bottleneck to progress. Don't wait too long, though, because small changes in trajectory compound over time. The earlier projects are funded, the bigger the impact.

Fortunately, the momentum is already building. More startups and funds are explicitly anti-aging. Large markets and lower risk are attracting entrepreneurs and investors alike. With enough pressure, a new therapeutic paradigm may arrive sooner than expected, so long as the R&D we invest in pays off.

Research and Development

If you're drawn to research, there's no shortage of work to be done. There are potential research opportunities in cryobiology, transplantation, gene circuits, and delivery systems for almost every therapeutic approach.

Better tools matter too. New animal models, organoids, clocks, and biomarkers can accelerate validation. Even just organizing or creating public databases and shared infrastructure can improve collaboration.

AI offers another advantage. Automated literature review, experiment design, and molecular modeling could dramatically speed progress. Embodied AI that can control robots could take on work in the physical world as well.

Rather than developing therapies directly, you could build tools and platforms that enable others to do so. However, platform choice matters. Improving small-molecule screening in model organisms, for example, may have limited impact given poor translation to humans and the known limits of small molecules. Platforms should support approaches with real potential for lifespan extension.

If you prefer to focus on building, choose areas that align with both your skills and the highest impact opportunities.

Biostasis needs help across many fronts, especially in marketing. Increasing adoption may be the single most urgent task. Operations, field work, cryoprotectants, and rewarming technologies also need development. Progress here is largely a matter of effort and funding. There are hundreds of new cryoprotectants and protocols waiting to be tested, and it only takes one breakthrough to make the next leap forward in cryopreservation.

Replacement strategies also offer many options for new ventures. We need ways to make cells reproduce like rabbits, prevent infighting between donor and patient organs, and get organs into and out of the body. The most urgent help is needed on the supply side, but robotics will be critical as organ availability scales beyond human surgical capacity.

Bioengineering and gene therapy platforms also offer many entry points. Some areas are overfunded, while others are understaffed. Look for neglected but high-potential problems, such as gene delivery or extracellular matrix rejuvenation.

You could also build infrastructure for translating discoveries into therapies or operating contract research organizations. On the care side, longevity clinics, digital health platforms, and at-home diagnostics could improve access and adoption.

Key Takeaways

Decide who you are optimizing for. Think about the oldest person you care about and what it would take to save them. If you can save them, you can likely save everyone who matters to you. Let that goal guide your choices.

You don't need to do everything, and you don't need to work alone. Contribute where you can, collaborate with others, and adjust as you learn. Pace yourself. This is a long game, and sustained effort is what will ultimately matter.

There's no single correct path. You only need one that works for you, and you must pursue it seriously. Whether you aim to save one person or millions, clarity of purpose sustains motivation and maximizes impact. So while you don't need to know exactly what to do, commit to doing something. That will help put you in the right frame of mind for making progress. Attitude is everything.

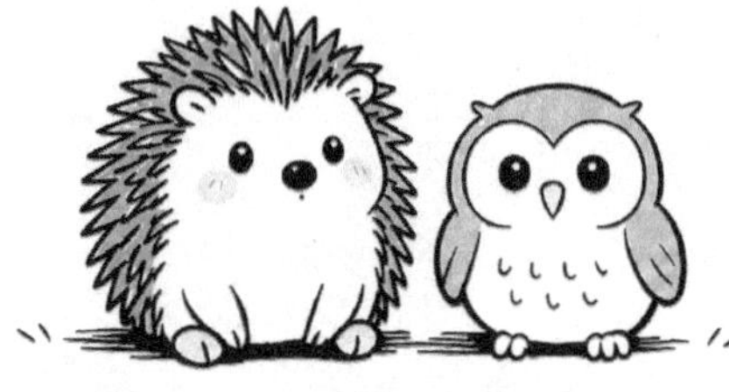

Sunday	Monday	Tuesday	Wednesday	Thursday	Friday	Saturday
				1 Solve aging	2 Solve aging	3 Solve aging
4 Solve aging	5 Solve aging	6 Solve aging	7 Solve aging	8 Solve aging	9 Solve aging	10 Solve aging
11 Solve aging	12 Solve aging	13 Solve aging	14 Solve aging	15 Solve aging	16 Solve aging	17 Solve aging
18 Solve aging	19 Solve aging	20 Solve aging	21 Solve aging	22 Solve aging	23 Solve aging	24 Solve aging
25 Solve aging	26 Solve aging	27 Solve aging	28 Solve aging	29 Solve aging	30 Solve aging	

CHAPTER 12

LONGEVITY MINDSET

People should be able to live as long as they like. This isn't the current state of affairs, but it's possible. If you want to bring it about, it will help you to adopt a pro-longevity mindset. This is more than a love of life or a fear of death. It means integrating certain ideas into the way you think and feel. Some of the ideas are big—bigger than our somewhat limited human intelligence can easily grasp. But if we take the time to recognize them and see how they relate to the mission, then these ideas can help us power through the work that needs to be done.

The most important mental shift is to admit that you have a problem —a deadly serious one. As things stand, aging limits every human life. Yours included.

It's valuable to occasionally embrace the pain of existential dread as a source of motivation. Too much might be counterproductive, as it may lead to depression and a sense of hopelessness. However, a little jolt of terror every now and then can help us focus. It can bring into perspective what matters and what doesn't. Many of life's problems seem much less daunting after reflecting on the total annihilation that awaits us.

Of course, this isn't a normal thing to do. The most common reaction to existential fear is denial. For most of human history, this was the best way to deal with the problem, and we have constructed elaborate psychological and social barriers to protect ourselves. Unfortunately, as we transition to a level of technology that allows us to solve the problem, this denial manifests in ways that slow progress toward solutions. Fortunately, mortal terror can motivate us to find a solution to death. Such a quixotic course of action is considered insane now, but will eventually be heralded as the greatest achievement of the human species.

Use this to your advantage by occasionally facing mortality head-on. Picture, briefly, a future in which no solution arrives in time: your life, and the lives of the people you love, simply end. Sit with that, then turn it into resolve to act—before it's too late. Remember: the best time to plant a tree was 20 years ago. The second best time is right now.

If you ever get caught up spending time on trivialities, or worrying about problems that are small in the grand scheme of things, a little reminder of, or meditation on, your big problem will help put them into perspective. From that point of view, you'll make better decisions about how to pursue radical life extension.

Fear can be a great motivator, but it isn't enough to maximize your productivity and chances of success. Everyone should also hang a carrot in front of themselves to go along with the stick. Fortunately, radical life extension provides a big carrot. So big that it's essentially inconceivable to our brains.

The value of an infinite lifespan is so huge that human minds aren't equipped to understand it. As an analogy, think of investing money. If you put money into an investment now, you get more money later. It's worth the upfront sacrifice to get a little bit more than you had. People routinely invest $1,000 to get $1,050 the next year.

However, with longevity, you invest effort and money to get more time. If your investment allows you to reach an indefinite lifespan, the payoff is so enormous that it would be worth great personal sacrifice now.

It's understandable that if you knew you were going to die, you might want to have a little fun while you're alive. But if cutting out junk food, exercising, and working tirelessly on longevity can get you an extra thousand years, then having less fun now will lead to many lifetimes of fun later.

The point isn't that we should all become robots that sacrifice everything in the pursuit of radical life extension. Human psychology doesn't work like that; we should all take breaks and find enjoyment along the way. The point is that the stakes are high; so, even if it's difficult to understand how high they truly are, we should use them to help push us to do our best.

It's not uncommon for the heat death of the universe to come up in conversations about longevity. That's a good thing if you want to personally witness how things go down. It's a bad thing, however, if it makes you feel like life extension is pointless because the universe has an expiration date.

It's important to recognize that the heat death of the universe doesn't matter. First, you have a more pressing problem. Second, it's farther away than humans can comprehend. Stars are still forming within our galaxy, and stars last a long time. Think about how old the universe is—about 14 billion years. Nobody can conceive of how long that is. It might as well be forever. If longevity technology could get you only a million years, that would be incredible. If it could get you the entire history of the universe so far—about 14 billion years—that would be unimaginable. But the heat death of the universe is so far away that cosmologists estimate it will occur on the order of 10^{100} years in the future. The universe is just getting started. With about 14 billion years behind us and tens of trillions of years of starlight ahead, there's a lot to look forward to. And who knows what tricks we'll come up with in the meantime.

More importantly, the heat death of the universe isn't something we can control. So it doesn't make sense to worry about it. Worrying about things you can't control will distract you from problems you can do something about, like aging. If you find yourself worrying about the long-term consequences of entropy, consider reading a bit about stoicism.

As the Stoics advised, you can develop self-control and fortitude to overcome destructive emotions. They emphasize focusing on what you can control rather than worrying about things that you can do nothing about. For example, you can control your own thoughts, actions, and reactions, so it makes sense to consider what to do about them. You can't control external events and other people's actions, so you should take them as a given. Adhering to this principle can help you achieve a tranquil and resilient state of mind, free from unnecessary worry. It also reserves your time and energy for plans and actions that can have an effect on the world.

For many years, the stoic thing to do about death was to accept it and move on with your life. Aging, fortunately, is now entering the realm of the controllable. So it finally makes sense to worry about it, to find ways to control it, and to put another nail in its coffin.

This applies to many things in life. Don't fret about everything you read about in the news. Don't worry about whether you will be bored on your 300th birthday. Focus on the things you can control and the steps you can take toward advancing longevity technology.

By concentrating on the main problem and the things you can do to help solve it, you will be much more effective. Focus is how hard problems get solved. By relentlessly pursuing a goal, being determined, and leveraging all of your resourcefulness, you'll have the best chance at changing the way the future plays out.

Remember, the future is bright. One day there will be a generation that doesn't feel helpless in the face of mortality. They won't see their friends and family grow old and die. Death will be an external problem, a tragedy, not an intrinsic part of their existence to be confused with the joys of life. There will be other things to fear, like crime or natural disasters, but people won't be trapped in a sealed room, waiting for the air to run out.

The longevity movement will eventually end and, not too far in the future, people will just live. An unimaginably long life will just be life, and the idea of extending it won't mean anything. People won't have to experience mortal terror, at least not in the same way that people today go through it. There won't be a pressing need for any additional work on the human body. Work will go on, and people will likely develop many biological and artificial improvements but, with aging solved, people may choose to simply enjoy their eternal youth.

Getting there is a journey through unknown territory that will require mental, emotional, and physical fortitude. It's both a moral imperative and an enormous opportunity. To give it your all, acknowledge the problem, visualize the rewards of solving it, avoid distractions, and focus on what you can control. Work on the things you can do each day to make a difference. If you want your life to persist, then be persistent in maximizing your chances by keeping an eye on the prize and hope in your heart.

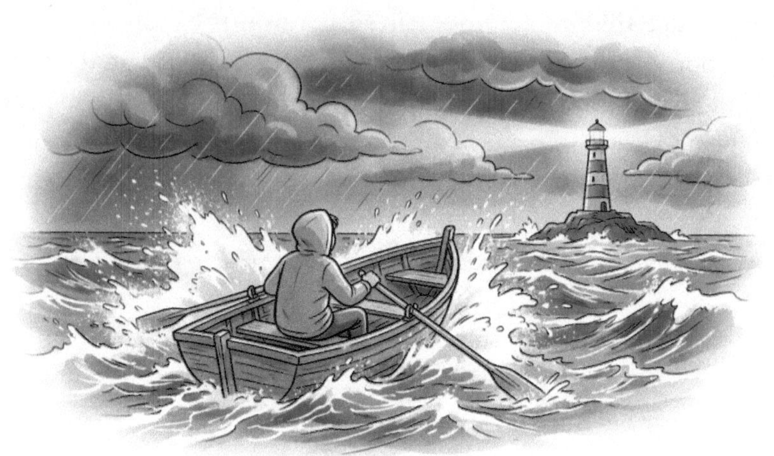

CHAPTER 13

REASONS FOR HOPE

In the past, there was no way to solve aging. Today, there is hope.

The biggest reason for hope is simple: you are still alive. While you're here, you have a chance. Not only a chance that something will happen, but also a chance to make something happen. You can place some bets and play some cards because, while you're alive, you can influence the course of history. You may be unable to solve the problem of aging on your own, but you don't have to. That's because the second reason for hope is that you aren't alone.

Thousands are working to bring radical life extension to everyone who wants it—engineers, scientists, investors, medical professionals, communicators, and more. They are some of the smartest, bravest, and kindest people you will ever meet. If you're working toward a solution to aging, then they are all on your team.

We're a team that's working on something more awesome than rocket ships, more valuable than blockchains, and more revolutionary than artificial intelligence. It's a group of people trying to save billions of lives. Normally, that only happens in movies, but it's happening right now, and you can be a part of it.

What's more, the team is growing. Every day, new people learn about the longevity field. This small but determined network is building, investing, and spreading the word. Talent and capital are trickling in. Before too long, there will be a flood.

The third reason for hope is that we aren't starting from zero. Decades of work have already gone into modern longevity research and development. We're now seeing the benefits of the early efforts toward understanding aging and designing therapies. Once these technologies come of age, the physical decline we currently associate with the passing of years will vanish. Age really will be just a number.

Bioengineering has produced first-generation therapies that are currently going through clinical trials and should be available soon. Many more are in development, and waves of new technology will begin to create longer and healthier lives. Moreover, some of the biggest problems in bioengineering are beginning to show cracks. As gene therapy delivery and gene circuit design become easier, safer, and more effective, there will be an explosion of options for treating age-related disease, and these chronic conditions will begin to bite the dust.

Even before then, therapeutic replacement will take a shortcut around drug development. Delivering young replacement parts will not only cure many diseases, but also reverse the underlying damage that causes aging.

Furthermore, biostasis is already here. While still unproven, existing evidence suggests that even the rudimentary biostasis technology used decades ago may save the lives of those who chose to employ it, and the technology is only getting better. Thousands have already decided not to give up when their biological clocks run out. With luck, millions more will follow in their footsteps. Good things come to those who wait, but only if they wait in biostasis.

The final reason for hope is that now you know. You know what is at stake. Even though your own personal hourglass has a bit less sand at the top than it did before, now you can make every remaining grain count.

Connect with the longevity community and begin to dedicate some of your time to it. We know your time is valuable. Spend it wisely. Spend it with us, working on what really matters. Not a legacy or a footnote in history, but the opportunity for a real happily-ever-after for you, your family, your friends, and, eventually, the whole human race.

Glossary

Aging is the gradual accumulation of diverse damage throughout the body.

Bioengineering is a strategy for understanding and modifying human biology to slow and reverse aging.

Biostasis is pausing biological processes through low temperatures, chemical fixation, or both.

Bodyoid is a lab-grown body intentionally lacking the brain structures that could give rise to a mind.

Chemopreservation is the use of chemical fixatives to preserve cells, tissues, and organs.

Cryogenics is the discipline of producing cold temperatures.

Cryonics is a strategy for preserving a patient's body with cold temperatures until medical technology advances enough to help them.

Cryopreservation is the use of cold temperatures to preserve cells, tissues, and organs.

Dewar is an insulated, vacuum-sealed container designed for cryopreserving things in liquid nitrogen.

Ectogenesis is growing organisms or tissue constructs in an artificial womb.

Epigenetics is the system that controls which genes are expressed.

Extracellular matrix is the structural scaffold produced by cells that shapes your body.

Gene therapy is a technology for altering the DNA and RNA inside a cell.

Healthspan is the length of time you are healthy during your life, currently averaging about 60 years.

Lifespan is the length of time you are alive, currently averaging about 80 years.

Longevity escape velocity is when technology reverses aging damage as quickly as it occurs.

Partial reprogramming is resetting the epigenetics of a cell without changing cell type.

Replacement is a strategy for substituting functional body components for ones that are diseased, damaged, or lost.

Additional Resources

Websites

longbiofellowship.org - The most hardcore anti-aging organization in the world.

vitalismfoundation.org - The strategic network to solve aging and death.

agingbiotech.info - The open database of longevity resources.

fightaging.org - Longevity science blog covering the latest news and research.

Books

Human Cryopreservation Procedures by Aschwin de Wolf and Charles Platt

Replacing Aging by Jean Hébert

Molecular Biology of the Cell by Bruce Alberts

Immune by Philipp Dettmer

Regenesis by George Church and Ed Regis

How Not to Age by Michael Greger

Do You Believe in Magic? by Paul Offit

Why We Sleep by Matthew Walker

Exercised by Daniel Lieberman

Resilient by Rick Hanson

A Guide to the Good Life by William B. Irvine

Acknowledgments

I would like to thank everyone in the longevity community for their hard work and dedication.

Thanks to the Longevity Biotech Fellowship for creating the Longevity Acceleration Roadmap, on which this book is based.

Special thanks to Mark Hamalainen and Nathan Cheng for their mentorship and undying support.

Beta-readers
Simon Franek, Tim Borer, David Lertola

Expert Review
Mark Hamalainen, Micah Zoltu, Anastasia Egorova, Karl Pfleger, Eli Mohamad, Seth Paulson, Reason, Borys Wrobel, Adam Gries, Alex Plesa

Editing
Hugh Barker, Andrew Lockett, Emily Price Soli, Mark Hamalainen

Artwork
Cat Thu Nguyen Huu

Attribution
Metabolism diagram modified from: https://commons.wikimedia.org/wiki/File:Human_Metabolism_-_Pathways.jpg by Evans Love; License: https://creativecommons.org/licenses/by-sa/4.0/deed.en

About the Author

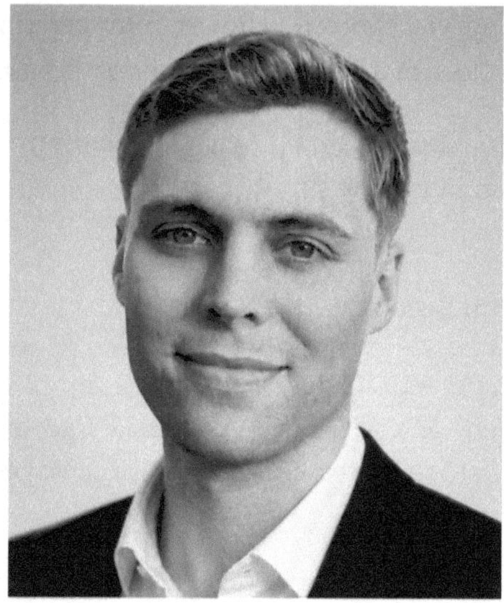

Kris studied engineering at Carnegie Mellon University and the University of Pennsylvania. He is an entrepreneur with a background in robotics, artificial intelligence, and software engineering, and an angel investor in companies developing longevity biotechnology.

For more information, please visit krisborer.com